The Medical Book of Lists:
A Primer of Differential Diagnosis in Internal Medicine

The Medical Book of Lists:
A Primer of Differential Diagnosis in Internal Medicine

Norton J. Greenberger, M.D.
Peter T. Bohan Professor of Medicine
Department of Medicine
Kansas University Medical Center

Alexander Davis, M.D.
Formerly Chief Resident in Medicine
Kansas University Medical Center

Roger Dreiling, M.D.
Formerly Chief Resident in Medicine
Kansas University Medical Center

YEAR BOOK MEDICAL PUBLISHERS, INC.
Chicago • London

Library of Congress Cataloging of Publication Data

Greenberger, Norton J., 1933–
    The medical book of lists.

    1. Diagnosis, Differential—Case studies.
I. Davis, Alexander.   II. Dreiling, Roger.   III. Title.
[DNLM: 1. Diagnosis, Differential—Handbooks.
WB   141.5   G798m]
RC71.5.G7   1983   616.07′5   83–10604
ISBN 0–8151–3939–X

Preface

Two of the most important considerations in the practice of internal medicine are the formulation of the differential diagnosis and the recognition of precise criteria upon which to base a specific diagnosis. We have written this book because we believe that there is need for a reasonably brief treatise that deals primarily with differential diagnosis. The book is a direct outgrowth of morning report sessions at the University of Kansas Medical Center. At these sessions, cases are presented as unknowns and resident physicians are asked to develop a differential diagnosis and also to indicate the specific criteria necessary to establish various diagnoses. This book, which contains over 230 lists, is a selective distillation of topics covered at morning report exercises. As such, the book is not a substitute for standard textbooks of medicine. Rather, it is viewed as a quick reference to key questions that may arise on ward rounds or at conferences.

Several individuals have contributed greatly to this book. We thank several former chief residents and are especially indebted to our secretaries, Juanita Stika, Mrs. Shirley Sears, Mrs. Patty Wiens, and Mrs. Jane Hollander for their preparation of the manuscript.

Norton J. Greenberger, M.D.
Alexander Davis, M.D.
Roger Dreiling, M.D.

TABLE OF CONTENTS

I—Cardiology

I-1 INNOCENT MURMURS

I. Patients in whom innocent murmurs are more likely to occur
   A. Children and adolescents
   B. Pregnant women
   C. Anxious persons
   D. Funnel-breasted or flat-chested persons
   E. Persons with the straight-back syndrome
   F. Hyperthyroid and anemic persons
II. Types of innocent murmurs
   Innocent murmurs may be classified as follows:
   A. Completely innocent
      1. Cervical venous hum
      2. Supraclavicular arterial bruit
      3. Still's murmur
      4. Mammary souffle
      5. Ejection systolic murmur in the pulmonary area
      6. Innocent abdominal murmurs
   B. Relatively innocent
      1. Early systolic murmur
      2. Pulmonary systolic murmur with high output states
         (hemic murmur)

I-2 CAUSES OF EXPIRATORY SPLITTING OF SECOND HEART SOUND

   I. Atrial septal defect (little respiratory variation)
   II. Pulmonary stenosis (diminished P_2; respiratory variation)
   III. Right bundle branch block (respiratory variation)
   IV. Mitral insufficiency (uncommon with heart failure)
   V. Ventricular septal defect (difficult to appreciate clinically)
   VI. Pulmonary hypertension, especially thromboembolic (often close
       and fixed splitting with accentuated P_2)
   VII. Postoperative atrial septal defect (respiratory variation)
   VIII. Sickle cell anemia (respiratory variation)
   IX. Idiopathic dilation of pulmonary artery (respiratory variation)
   X. Normal adolescence (in recumbent posture)
   XI. Wolff-Parkinson-White syndrome (occasional case)
   XII. Pulmonary valvular insufficiency
   XIII. Straight back syndrome
   XIV. Right ventricular decompensation (occasional case)
   XV. Left ventricular paced or ectopic beats

I-3 CAUSES OF SINGLE SECOND HEART SOUND

   I. Tetralogy of Fallot
   II. Truncus and pseudotruncus arteriosus
   III. Very severe pulmonary valvular stenosis (occasional case)
   IV. Tricuspid atresia
   V. Aortic stenosis (occasional case)
   VI. Left bundle branch block (occasional case)
   VII. Age over 45 years (variable)

I-4 CAUSES OF CONTINUOUS THORACIC MURMURS

   I. Patent ductus arteriosus
   II. Coronary arteriovenous fistula
   III. Ruptured aortic sinus of Valsalva aneurysm
   IV. Aortic septal defect
   V. Ventricular septal defect and aortic insufficiency
   VI. Cervical venous hum
   VII. Anomalous left coronary artery
   VIII. Anomalous pulmonary artery
   IX. Mammary souffle
   X. Pulmonary arterial branch stenosis
   XI. Bronchial collateral circulation
   XII. Small atrial septal defect with mitral stenosis or atresia

I-5 MECHANISMS OF CONTINUOUS MURMURS

   I. Turbulent flow within veins, e.g., the cervical venous hum, caput medusae about the umbilicus. These venous continuous murmurs have diastolic accentuation, whereas the remaining four groups display systolic accentuation.
   II. Communication between a systemic artery and a systemic vein, the right heart, or the pulmonary artery, e.g., systemic arteriovenous fistula, patent ductus arteriosus, aortic aneurysm rupture into the right heart.
   III. Severe narrowing of a systemic artery or a pulmonary artery, e.g., carotid artery stenosis, pulmonary arterial branch stenosis or thromboembolism.
   IV. Communication between pulmonary artery and vein: pulmonary arteriovenous fistula.
   V. Communication between left and right atrium, especially with a high left atrial pressure.

I-6 JONES CRITERIA (REVISED) FOR DIAGNOSIS OF ACUTE RHEUMATIC FEVER (RF)

I. Major manifestations
   A. Carditis
   B. Polyarthritis
   C. Chorea
   D. Erythema marginatum
   E. Subcutaneous nodules
II. Minor manifestations
   A. Fever
   B. Arthralgias
   C. Previous RF or RHD
   D. Elevated ESR or CRP
   E. Prolonged PR interval

Plus: Supporting evidence of preceding streptococcal infection: history of scarlet fever; (+) culture group A streptococcus pharyngitis, increased strep. antibodies. American Heart Association, 1965

I-7 CAUSES OF MITRAL REGURGITATION

I. Spontaneous rupture of chordae tendinae
II. Trauma
III. Mitral valve prolapse
IV. Ischemia
V. Myocardial infarction
VI. Aneurysm of left ventricle involving the mitral annulus
VII. Infective endocarditis
VIII. Congestive cardiomyopathies
IX. IHSS
X. Rheumatic heart disease
XI. S.L.E.
XII. Scleroderma
XIII. Takayasu's arteritis
XIV. Myxomatous degeneration of mitral valve leaflets
XV. Calcified mitral annulus
XVI. Marfan's syndrome
XVII. Ehlers-Danlos syndrome
XVIII. Pseudoxanthoma elasticum
XIX. Ankylosing spondylitis

I-8 CAUSES OF AORTIC REGURGITATION
   I. Hypertension
   II. Infective endocarditis involving the aortic valve
   III. Dissecting thoracic aortic aneurysm
   IV. Trauma
   V. Rheumatic heart disease
   VI. Syphilis
   VII. Ankylosing spondylitis
   VIII. Rheumatoid arthritis
   IX. Takayasu's arteritis
   X. Reiter's syndrome
   XI. S.L.E.
   XII. Polychondritis
   XIII. Congenital (Marfan, Ehlers-Danlos, Pseudoxanthoma, osteogenesis imperfecta, mucopolysaccharidoses)
   XIV. Myxomatous degeneration of the valve
   XV. Ruptured sinus of valsalva aneurysm

I-9 CAUSES OF TRICUSPID REGURGITATION
   I. Rheumatic heart disease
   II. Endocarditis
   III. Myocardial infarction
   IV. Trauma
   V. Pulmonary hypertension
   VI. Ebstein's anomaly
   VII. Endocardial pacemaker wire
   VIII. Pulmonary artery catheter (Swan-Ganz®)

I-10 CLASSIFICATION OF ATRIAL SEPTAL DEFECTS
   I. Patent foramen ovale
   II. Persistent ostium secundum defect (fossa ovalis defect)
   III. Sinus venosus defect (proximal defect)
   IV. Endocardial cushion defect (complete and partial atrioventricular canal)
      A. Ostium primum defect (incomplete persistent common atrioventricular canal)
      B. Complete persistent common atrioventricular canal

I-11 COMPLICATIONS OF MITRAL STENOSIS

  I. Unrelated to severity of stenosis
   A. Atrial fibrillation
   B. Infective endocarditis
   C. Embolism
 II. Related to severity of stenosis
   A. Pulmonary edema
   B. Hemoptysis
   C. Dyspnea on exertion
   D. Pulmonary hypertension
   E. Right ventricular failure
III. Chest x-ray findings in mitral stenosis
   A. Enlargement of left atrium
   B. Enlargement of right ventricle
   C. Kerley B lines
   D. Enlargement of the pulmonary artery
   E. Cephalization of the pulmonary vasculature
   F. Calcification in the area of the mitral valve

I-12 RISK FACTORS FOR ATHEROSCLEROTIC HEART DISEASE

   I. Hypercholesterolemia
  II. Hypertension
 III. Smoking history
  IV. Diabetes mellitus (abnormal glucose tolerance)
   V. Family history of atherosclerosis (M.I., stroke, peripheral vascular disease)
  VI. Obesity
 VII. Sedentary living
VIII. Type A personality
  IX. Oral contraceptive use
   X. Chronic obstructive lung disease
  XI. Chronic renal failure
 XII. Hypertriglyceridemia (Type IV)

I-13 PURPOSES OF ECG EXERCISE TESTS

ECG exercise tests may be performed for the following reasons:

I. Screening an asymptomatic population
   A. For prognostic evaluation, e.g., in general epidemiology surveys or of insurance applicants
   B. For investigations of groups at high risk for coronary disease, e.g., hyperlipidemic patients
   C. For study of workers in critical positions, e.g., commercial aircraft pilots, military pilots
II. For diagnostic evaluation of patients with chest pain not typical of angina pectoris
III. For evaluating the degree of ischemia in patients with known angina or previous infarction - with regard to prognosis, treatment, permitted exercise level
IV. For evaluating therapeutic procedures in patients with angina, e.g., coronary artery bypass grafting or trial of new drugs
V. For evaluating severity of other lesions, e.g., aortic stenosis in children, mitral stenosis (there is a general reluctance to exercise adults with aortic stenosis for fear of provoking ventricular arrhythmias)
VI. For evaluating work capacity, e.g., following cardiac infarction
VII. To evaluate entry into or the results of rehabilitation or exercise training programs
VIII. To evaluate patients suspected of AV block or sinus node dysfunction

I-14 MYOCARDIAL INFARCTION: CLINICAL & HEMODYNAMIC SUBSETS

I. Class I
   A. Clinical: No evidence of heart failure
   B. Hemodynamic: PCWP = NML; CI > 2.2
   C. Prognosis: In hospital mortality 5-7%

II. Class II
   A. Clinical: Tachycardia, bibasilar rales to scapula tip and/or S_3 gallop
   B. Hemodynamic: PCWP > 18 mm Hg; CI > 2.2
   C. Prognosis: In hospital mortality 10-15%

III. Class III
   A. Clinical: Tachycardia, rales above tip of scapula, S_3 gallop or frank pulmonary edema
   B. Hemodynamic: PCWP ≤ 18; CI < 2.2
   C. Prognosis: In hospital mortality 25-50%

IV. Class IV (cardiogenic shock)
   A. Clinical: Hypotension, cool clammy extremities, mental confusion, decreased urine output
   B. Hemodynamic: PCWP > 18; CI < 2.2
   C. Prognosis: In hospital mortality 80-90%

References: Killip, T., III and Kimball, J.T.: Treatment of myocardial infarction in a coronary care unit. Am. J. Cardiol. 20:457,1967.

Forrester, J. and Waters, D.: Hospital treatment of congestive heart failure: Management according to hemodynamic profile. Am. J. Med. 65:173, 1978.

PCWP = Pulmonary capillary wedge pressure (mm Hg)
CI = Cardiac index (L/min/M^2)

I-15 PROGNOSTIC DETERMINANTS IN ISCHEMIC HEART DISEASE

   I. Objective severity of ischemia
      A. Duration of treadmill
      B. Degree of ST depression
  II. Degree of left ventricular dysfunction
 III. Recurrent ischemic events
      A. Myocardial infarction
      B. Unstable angina
      C. Cardiac sudden death
  IV. Extent of coronary atherosclerosis
   V. Others
      A. History of hypertension
      B. History of congestive heart failure
      C. Cardiomegaly on chest x-ray
      D. EKG abnormalities
         1. Ventricular arrhythmias
         2. Conduction defects
      E. Smoking

I-16 PSEUDOINFARCTION ECG PATTERNS

   I. Myocardial replacement
      A. Tumor
      B. Abscess
      C. Amyloid disease
      D. Pseudohypertrophic muscular dystrophy
  II. Nonmyocardial replacement
      A. Anatomic factors
         1. Emphysema
         2. Pneumothorax
 III. Depolarization abnormalities
      A. IHSS
      B. WPW syndrome
      C. LBBB
  IV. Right ventricular hypertrophy
      A. Cor pulmonale
      B. Mitral stenosis
   V. Left ventricular disease
      A. Left ventricular hypertrophy
      B. Congestive cardiomyopathy
  VI. Arrhythmias
      A. Ventricular tachycardia
      B. Electronic pacing of right ventricle
 VII. Congestive cardiomyopathy

IHSS = Idiopathic hypertrophic subaortic stenosis
WPW = Wolff-Parkinson-White
LBBB = Left bundle branch block

I-17 CAUSES OF SUDDEN, NONTRAUMATIC DEATH

I. Cardiac
  A. Atherosclerotic coronary artery disease
  B. Stokes-Adams syndrome
  C. Valvular heart disease
    1. Aortic stenosis
    2. Mitral valve prolapse
  D. Myocarditis
  E. Acute pericardial tamponade
  F. Primary myocardial disease
  G. Congestive heart disease
  H. Prolonged Q-T interval syndromes
  I. Drug effects
    1. Hypokalemia
    2. Digitalis
    3. Quinidine and other type I antiarrhythmics
    4. Tricyclic antidepressants
II. Pulmonary
  A. Cor pulmonale
    1. Acute
    2. Chronic
  B. Status asthmaticus
  C. Asphyxia
    1. Cafe coronary
III. Extracardiac
  A. Dissecting aortic aneurysm
  B. Exsanguinating hemorrhage
  C. Cerebrovascular accident
IV. Miscellaneous
  A. Sudden infant death syndrome
  B. Acute pancreatitis
  C. Unexplained

I-18 RISK FACTORS FOR ANTICOAGULATION

I. Pre-existing coagulation defect
II. Ulcerative lesion in the GI tract (P.U.D., U.C.)
III. Salicylate therapy
IV. Old age
V. Poor patient compliance
VI. Pregnancy
VII. Bacterial endocarditis
VIII. Liver disease
IX. Advanced retinopathy
X. Malignant hypertension

11

I-19 CARDIOMYOPATHY: PATHOLOGICAL CLASSIFICATION

I. Primary myocardial involvement
   A. Idiopathic
   B. Familial
   C. Alcoholic
   D. Peripartum
   E. Endocardial fibroelastosis
   F. Endomyocardial fibrosis
   G. Postcarditic
   H. Drugs (daunorubicin)
II. Secondary myocardial involvement
   A. Amyloidosis
   B. Hemochromatosis
   C. Sarcoidosis
   D. Connective tissue disease
      1. Lupus erythematosis
      2. Polyarteritis
      3. Scleroderma
      4. Dermatomyositis
   E. Neuromuscular disease
      1. Muscular dystrophy
      2. Myotonic dystrophy
      3. Friedreich's ataxia
      4. Refsum's disease
   F. Neoplastic
   G. Glycogen storage disease (Pompe's)
   H. Lipidoses
      1. Hunter-Hurler syndrome
      2. Fabry's disease
      3. Sandhoff's disease

Modified from: Glick, G. and Braunwald, E.: in *Harrison's Principles of Internal Medicine*, Isselbacher, K.J., Adams, R.D., Braunwald, E., Petersdorf, R.G., and Wilson, J.D. (eds.), 9th Edition, McGraw-Hill Book Company, New York City, 1980, p. 1142.

I-20 CONGESTIVE HEART FAILURE: PRECIPITATING CAUSES

    I. Pulmonary embolism
   II. Myocardial infarction
  III. Arrhythmias
  IV. Increasingly severe hypertension
   V. Noncompliance with medications
     A. Digitalis
     B. Diuretics
  VI. Excess dietary sodium
 VII. Excessive amounts of intravenous fluids
VIII. Drugs (See Table I-22)
     A. Propranolol and other beta blockers
     B. Cardiotoxic drugs
       1. Adriamycin
  IX. Pregnancy
   X. High output states with increased metabolic demands
     A. Fever
     B. Hyperthyroidism
     C. Anemia
     D. A-V fistula
 XII. Rheumatic and other forms of myocarditis

I-21 REVERSIBLE CAUSES OF CONGESTIVE HEART FAILURE

    I. Anemia
   II. Hyperthyroidism
  III. Atrial myxoma
  IV. Arteriovenous fistula
   V. Surgically correctable valvular heart disease
  VI. Surgically correctable congenital heart disease
 VII. Cardiac arrhythmias in an otherwise normal heart
VIII. Thiamine deficiency
  IX. Alcohol

I-22 DRUGS THAT MAY CAUSE DETERIORATION IN HEART FAILURE

I. Alcohol
II. Indomethacin (and other anti-inflammatory agents, e.g., ibuprofen)
III. Phenylbutazone
IV. Chlorpropamide
V. Inderal, other β-adrenergic blocking drugs
VI. Estrogens
VII. Androgens
VIII. Vasoconstrictors(?)
IX. Sodium retaining steroids (e.g., aldosterone)
X. Minoxidil
XI. Norpace
XII. Antineoplastic drugs (e.g. Adriamycin)
XIII. Tricyclic psychotrophic drugs (e.g. Nortriptyline)

From Podrid, PJ, et al. N Engl J Med 302:614, 1980

I-23 HYPERTENSION: DIFFERENTIAL DIAGNOSIS

I. Systolic and diastolic hypertension
  A. Primary (idiopathic)
  B. Secondary
    1. Renal
      a. Renal parenchymal disease
        (1) acute glomerulonephritis
        (2) chronic glomerulonephritis
        (3) polycystic disease
        (4) connective tissue diseases
        (5) diabetic nephropathy
        (6) hydronephrosis
      b. Renovascular disease
      c. Renin producing tumors
      d. Renoprival disease
      e. Primary Na retention (Liddle's syndrome, Gordon's syndrome)

2. Endocrine
    a. Acromegaly
    b. Hypothyroidism
    c. Adrenal
        (1) cortical
            (a) Cushing's syndrome
            (b) Primary aldosteronism
            (c) Congenital adrenal hyperplasia
        (2) medullary (pheochromocytoma)
    d. Extra-adrenal chromaffin tumors
    e. Hypercalcemia
    f. Exogenous
        (1) estrogen
        (2) glucocorticoid
        (3) mineralocorticoid (carbenoxolone, licorice, tobacco products)
        (4) sympathomimetics
        (5) MAO inhibitors with tyramine containing foods
3. Coarctation of the aorta
4. Pregnancy
5. Neurogenic
    a. Psychogenic
    b. Increased intracranial pressure
        (1) respiratory acidosis
        (2) encephalitis
        (3) brain tumor
    c. Lead poisoning
    d. Familial dysautonomia
    e. Acute porphyria
    f. Quadriplegia
    g. Postoperative
6. Miscellaneous
    a. Increased vascular volume
        (1) polycythemia vera
        (2) postoperative
    b. Burns
    c. Carcinoid syndrome

(continued)

I-23 HYPERTENSION: DIFFERENTIAL DIAGNOSIS (CONTINUED)

II. Systolic hypertension
   A. Increased cardiac output
      1. Aortic valvular regurgitation
      2. Arteriovenous fistula, patent ductus
      3. Thyrotoxicosis
      4. Paget's disease of bone
      5. Beriberi
      6. Hyperkinetic heart syndrome
      7. Anemia
   B. Rigidity of aorta

Adapted from: Kaplan, N.M.: in *Heart Disease. A Textbook of Cardiovascular Medicine*. E. Braunwald (Ed.), W.B. Saunders Co., Philadelphia, 1980, p. 881.

I-24 FACTORS INDICATING AN ADVERSE PROGNOSIS IN HYPERTENSION

I. Black race
II. Young age
III. Male
IV. Persistent diastolic BP > 115 mm Hg
V. Smoking
VI. Diabetes mellitus
VII. Hyperlipidemia
VIII. Obesity
IX. Evidence of end organ damage
   A. Cardiac
   B. Ophthalmologic
   C. Renal impairment
   D. Central nervous system: stroke

Modified from: Williams, G.H., et al.: in *Harrison's Principles of Internal Medicine*, Isselbacher, K.J., Adams, R.D., Braunwald, E., Petersdorf, R.G., and Wilson, J.D. (eds.), 9th Edition, McGraw-Hill Book Company, New York City, 1980, p. 1168.

I-25 CARDIOGENIC SYNCOPE

I. Disturbances of cardiac rhythm
  A. Complete AV block (Adams-Stokes attacks)
  B. Paroxysmal supraventricular tachycardia
  C. Extreme sinus bradycardia or transient sinus arrest (sick sinus syndrome)
  D. Ventricular slowing, tachycardia, or fibrillation without AV block
    1. Coronary artery disease
    2. Quinidine
    3. Aortic stenosis
    4. Congenital deafness with prolonged QT interval
    5. Mitral click-murmur syndrome
    6. Related to phenothiazines or digitalis
II. Aortic stenosis
  A. Valvular stenosis
  B. Discrete subvalvular stenosis
  C. Diffuse muscular subvalvular stenosis
III. Atrial myxoma or ball thrombus
IV. Congenital heart disease
  A. Tetralogy of Fallot-pulmonary stenosis
  B. Eisenmenger's complex
V. Idiopathic or thromboembolic pulmonary hypertension
VI. Coronary artery disease (myocardial infarction and angina pectoris)
VII. Pericarditis
VIII. Dissecting aortic aneurysm

I-26 CAUSES OF SYNCOPE

I. Vasodepressor (vasovagal)
II. Cardiogenic
III. Carotid sinus
IV. Posttussive
V. Postmicturition
VI. Orthostatic hypotension
VII. Miscellaneous
  A. Carcinoid syndrome
  B. Pregnancy
  C. Hysteria
VIII. Carotid and vertebrobasilar artery disease, aortic arch syndrome
IX. Pulmonary embolism

I-27 PERICARDITIS

I. Infectious pericarditis
   A. Viral
   B. Pyogenic
   C. Tuberculous
   D. Mycotic
   E. Other infections (syphilis, parasitic)
II. Non-infectious pericarditis
   A. Acute myocardial infarction
   B. Uremia
   C. Neoplastic
      1. Primary tumors (benign or malignant)
      2. Tumors metastatic to pericardium
   D. Myxedema
   E. Cholesterol
   F. Chylopericardium
   G. Trauma
   H. Aortic aneurysm (with pericardial sac leakage)
   I. Postirradiation
   J. Associated with atrial septal defect
   K. Associated with severe chronic anemia
   L. Infectious mononucleosis
   M. Familial Mediterranean fever
   N. Familial pericarditis
   O. Sarcoidosis
   P. Acute idiopathic
III. Pericarditis presumably related to hypersensitivity or autoimmunity
   A. Rheumatic fever
   B. Collagen vascular disease
      1. Systemic lupus erythematosis
      2. Rheumatoid arthritis
      3. Scleroderma
   C. Drug-induced
      1. Procainamide
      2. Hydralazine
      3. Other
   D. Post-cardiac injury
      1. Post-myocardial infarction (Dressler's syndrome)
      2. Post-pericardiotomy

Modified from: Braunwald, E.: in *Harrison's Principles of Internal Medicine*, Isselbacher, K.J., Adams, R.D., Braunwald, E., Petersdorf, R.G., and Wilson, J.D. (eds.), 9th Edition, McGraw-Hill Book Company, New York City, 1980, p. 1150.

I-28 ETIOLOGY OF CHRONIC CONSTRICTIVE PERICARDITIS

    I. Unknown
    II. Following idiopathic pericarditis
    III. Specific infection
        A. Bacterial
        B. Tuberculosis (50% - 65% of treated pericarditis)
        C. Fungal disease (rare): histoplasmosis, coccidioidomycosis
        D. Viral disease, esp. Coxsackie B_3
        E. Parasitic disease: amebiasis, echinococcosis
    VI. Connective tissue disease: rheumatoid arthritis, lupus erythematosus
    V. Neoplastic disease
        A. Primary mesothelioma
        B. Secondary lymphoma, bronchogenic carcinoma
    VI. Trauma
        A. Blunt or penetrating
        B. Surgical (rare)
    VII. Radiation therapy
    VIII. Uremic
    IX. Hereditary (mulibrey nanism—Finland)

I-29 CLINICAL FEATURES OF CONSTRICTIVE PERICARDITIS (137 cases)*

    I. Symptoms
        A. Effort dyspnea—89.8%
        B. Chest pain—24.1%†
        C. RUQ or epigastric pain—10.9%
        D. Effort syncope—4
        E. Orthopnea, paroxysmal nocturnal dyspnea—3

*Wychulis et al. J Thorac Cardiovasc Surg 62:608, 1971

†Most studies do not report so high a prevalence of chest pain. Hirschmann. Am Heart J 96:111, 1978

    II. Physical findings
        A. Atrial fibrillation—27%
        B. Cervical veins engorged. Venous pressure 15-44 cm H_2O
        C. Liver enlarged—134 cases
        D. Ascites—77.4%
        E. Peripheral edema—61%
        F. Pleural effusion—47%
        G. Paradoxical pulse—29%
        H. Early diastolic heart sound—20 cases

I-30 ETIOLOGY OF PERICARDIAL EFFUSION

I. Serous
   A. Congestive heart failure
   B. Hypoalbuminemia
   C. Post-thoracic irradiation
   D. Recurrent viral pericarditis (also may be serosanguineous)
II. Serosanguineous
   A. Uremia
   B. Neoplastic pericarditis
   C. Traumatic pericarditis
III. Serofibrinous
   A. Bacterial pericarditis
   B. Tuberculous pericarditis
   C. Systemic erythematosis (also may be serous)
IV. Hemorrhagic
   A. Following cardiac surgery
   B. Myocardial infarction plus anticoagulants
   C. Traumatic pericarditis
   D. Vascular pericardial tumors
V. Chylous
   A. Idiopathic
   B. Following cardiac surgery
   C. Neoplastic pericarditis with lymphatic obstruction
   D. Lymph obstruction by intrathoracic masses
VI. Cholesterol
   A. Idiopathic
   B. Myxedema

Modified from: Darsee, J.R. and Braunwald, E.: in *Heart Disease: A Textbook of Cardiology Medicine*, W.B. Saunders Co., Philadelphia, 1980, p. 1537.

I-31 CAUSES OF CARDIAC TAMPONADE

I. Idiopathic pericarditis
II. Iatrogenic (diagnostic procedures, pacing, etc.)
III. Anticoagulants in idiopathic, uremic, malignant, and post-infarction pericarditis
IV. Rupture of the myocardium
V. Dissection of aortic aneurysm into pericardial sac
VI. Malignant pericarditis
VII. Trauma
VIII. Acute rheumatic fever
IX. Following cardiac operations

Modified from: Kennealey, G.T., et al.: in *Cancer: A Comprehensive Treatise*, Frederick F. Becker (Ed.), Plenum Press, New York, 1977, Vol. 5, p. 8.

I-32 CLASSIFICATION OF PULMONARY HYPERTENSION

I. Primary (essential or idiopathic)
II. Secondary
- A. Caused by reduction of the pulmonary vascular bed due to
  1. Pulmonary parenchymal disease: emphysema, granuloma, fibrosis
  2. Pulmonary arterial disease: thromboembolism, pulmonary arterial branch stenosis, parasitism
  3. Hypoxia and respiratory acidosis due to alveolar hypoventilation
- B. Caused by congenital left-to-right shunt
- C. Caused by increased pulmonary venous pressure due to
  1. Left ventricular failure
  2. Mitral stenosis, left atrial myxoma, cor triatriatum
  3. Pulmonary vein obstruction

I-33 PULMONARY DISORDERS PREDISPOSING TO COR PULMONALE

I. Intrinsic disease of the lungs and airways
- A. Chronic obstructive pulmonary disease
- B. Diffuse pulmonary interstitial disease
- C. Pulmonary vascular disease
II. Chest bellows malfunctions
- A. Neuromuscular diseases
- B. Obesity ("Pickwickian syndrome")
- C. Kyphoscoliosis
III. Inadequate respiratory drive
- A. Primary alveolar hypoventilation
- B. Chronic mountain sickness

Modified from: Fishman, A.P.: in *Harrison's Principles of Internal Medicine*, Isselbacher, K.J., Adams, R.D., Braunwald, E., Petersdorf, R.G., and Wilson, J.D. (eds.), 9th Edition, McGraw-Hill Book Company, New York City, 1980, p. 1136.

I-34 PULMONARY VALVULAR INSUFFICIENCY

I. Congenital
  A. With Tetralogy of Fallot
  B. With Eisenmenger's syndrome
  C. With Marfan's syndrome
  D. Isolated
  E. With patent ductus arteriosus
  F. With idiopathic dilation of the pulmonary artery
II. Acquired as a result of other congenital heart disease
  A. Following operation on the stenotic pulmonary valve
  B. With pulmonary hypertension related to patent ductus arteriosus, atrial septal defect, or ventricular septal defect
III. As a result of acquired heart disease
  A. With idiopathic or thromboembolic pulmonary hypertension
  B. With mitral stenosis
  C. With bacterial endocarditis
  D. With rheumatic fever
  E. With syphilis
  F. With carcinoid syndrome
  G. With aneurysm of the pulmonary artery (often syphilitic)
  H. With pulmonary hypertension and chronic lung disease

I-35 FACTORS PREDISPOSING TO THROMBOEMBOLISM

I. Heart disease, especially
  A. Myocardial infarction
  B. Atrial fibrillation
  C. Cardiomyopathy
  D. Congestive heart failure
II. Postoperative state, especially operations on abdomen or pelvis, splenectomy, and orthopedic procedures on lower extremities
III. Pregnancy and parturition
IV. Neoplastic disease
V. Polycythemia
VI. Prolonged immobilization
VII. Hemorrhage
VIII. Fractures, especially of the hip
IX. Obesity
X. Varicose veins
XI. Prior history of thromboembolic disease
XII. Certain drugs: oral contraceptives, estrogens
XIII. Following cerebrovascular accidents

I-36 DIGITALIS INTOXICATION

    I. Patients with increased risk of digitalis intoxication
- A. Renal insufficiency or failure
- B. Malabsorption
- C. Elderly patients
- D. Obese patients
- E. Electrolyte imbalance (decreased K+, increased Ca++)
- F. Liver disease (digitoxin only)
- G. Thyroid disease (hypothyroidism)
- H. Pulmonary disease

    II. Diagnosis of digitalis intoxication
- *A. Symptoms: diarrhea, anorexia, nausea, emesis, visual disturbances
- *B. Arrhythmias
- *C. Digitalis dose excessive for body weight
  - 1. Usual maintenance dose of digoxin is 3 μg/kg
- *D. Digitalis dose excessive in the presence of impaired renal function
- *E. Increased serum digitalis glycoside levels
- F. Improvement in items A, B, and E after discontinuation of and/or readjustment in glycoside dosage

*These findings are not always present.

II—Endocrinology-Metabolism

II-I DISORDERS ASSOCIATED WITH HYPOPITUITARISM

I. Primary
- A. Ischemic necrosis of the pituitary
  1. Postpartum (Sheehan's syndrome)
  2. Diabetes mellitus
  3. Other systemic diseases (temporal arteritis, sickle-cell disease and trait, arteriosclerosis, eclampsia)
- B. Pituitary tumors
  1. Primary intrasellar (chromophobe adenoma, craniopharyngioma)
  2. Parasellar (meningioma, optic nerve glioma)
- C. Aneurysm of intracranial internal carotid artery
- D. Pituitary apoplexy (almost always related to a primary pituitary tumor)
- E. Cavernous sinus thrombosis
- F. Infectious disease (tuberculosis, syphilis, malaria, meningitis, fungal disease)
- G. Infiltrative disease (hemochromatosis)
- H. Immunologic (associated with pernicious anemia, or subsequent to repeated injections of heterologous pituitary hormones)
- I. Iatrogenic
  1. Irradiation to nasopharynx
  2. Irradiation to sella
  3. Surgical destruction
- J. Primary empty sella syndrome
- K. Metabolic disorders (chronic renal failure)
- L. Idiopathic (frequently monohormonal and occasionally familial)

II. Secondary
- A. Destruction of pituitary stalk
  1. Trauma
  2. Compression by tumor or aneurysm
  3. Iatrogenic (surgical)

B. Hypothalamic or other central nervous system disease
1. Inflammatory (sarcoid)
2. Infiltrative (lipid storage diseases)
3. Trauma
4. Toxic (vincristine)
5. Hormone-induced (glucocorticoids, gonadal steroids)
6. Tumors (primary, metastatic, lymphomas, leukemia)
7. Idiopathic (frequently congenital or familial, often restricted to one or two hormones, and may be reversible)
8. Nutritional (starvation, obesity)
9. Anorexia nervosa
10. Psychosocial dwarfism
11. Pinealoma

Adapted from: Frohman, L.A.: in *Endocrinology and Metabolism*, Felig, P., Baxter, J.D., Broadus, A.E., and Frohman, L.A. (eds.), 1st Edition, McGraw-Hill Book Company, New York, 1981, p. 176.

II-2 DIFFERENTIAL DIAGNOSIS OF HYPERPROLACTINEMIA

I. Prolactin-secreting pituitary tumor
II. Pharmacologic agents
  A. Monoamine synthesis inhibitors (alpha-methyldopa)
  B. Monoamine depletors (reserpine)
  C. Dopamine receptor antagonists (phenothiazines, butyrophenones, thioxanthenes)
  D. Monoamine uptake inhibitors (tricyclic antidepressants)
  E. Estrogens (oral contraceptives)
  F. Narcotics (morphine, heroin)
III. Central nervous system disorders
  A. Inflammatory/infiltrative (sarcoidosis, histiocytosis)
  B. Traumatic (stalk section)
  C. Neoplastic (hypothalamic or parasellar tumors)
IV. Other
  A. Hypothyroidism
  B. Renal failure
  C. Cirrhosis
  D. Nonendocrine tumors with ectopic hormone production
  E. Chest wall diseases
  F. Spinal cord lesions
V. "Idiopathic hyperprolactinemia"

Adapted from: Frohman, L.A.: in *Endocrinology and Metabolism*, Felig, P., Baxter, J.D., Broadus, A.E., and Frohman, L.A. (eds.), 1st Edition, McGraw-Hill Book Company, New York, 1981, p. 209.

II-3 CLINICAL FEATURES OF ACROMEGALY

Clinical features
I. Enlargement of hands, feet, nose, jaw
II. Soft tissue overgrowth
III. Weight gain
IV. Amenorrhea
V. Decreased libido
VI. Arthritis
VII. Hypertrichosis
VIII. Hypertension
IX. Glucose intolerance
X. Cardiac arrhythmias
XI. Visual field defects
XII. Paresthesias/peripheral neuropathy
XIII. Carpal tunnel syndrome

Diagnosis
I. Inappropriately ↑ plasma growth hormone
II. Failure of IV glucose to suppress plasma growth hormone
III. Abnormal growth hormone response to thyrotropin releasing hormone
IV. Hyperglycemia and glucosuria
V. ↑ sella turcica (90%)
VI. Abnormal CT scan

II-4 FEATURES COMMONLY ASSOCIATED WITH THE PRIMARY EMPTY SELLA SYNDROME

	Frequency, %
Females	83.7
Obesity	78.4
Systemic hypertension	30.5
Benign intracranial hypertension (pseudotumor cerebri)	10.5
CSF rhinorrhea	9.7

Jordan et al.: The primary empty sella syndrome. Am J Med 62:569, 1977.

II-5 PHYSIOLOGICAL CLASSIFICATION OF GALACTORRHEA

I. Failure of normal hypothalamic inhibition of prolactin release
    A. Pituitary stalk section
    B. Drugs
    C. Central nervous system disease
II. Enhanced prolactin-releasing factor
    A. Hypothyroidism
III. Enhanced prolactin release independent of the normal inhibition and release mechanisms
    A. Pituitary tumors
        1. Prolactin-secreting tumors (Forbes-Albright syndrome)
        2. Mixed growth hormone and prolactin
    B. Ectopic production of human placental lactogen and prolactin
        1. Hydatidiform moles and chorioepitheliomas
        2. Others (bronchogenic carcinoma and hypernephroma)
IV. Idiopathic (following or not following pregnancy or contraceptions, with or without amenorrhea)

Modified from: Emerson, R. and Wilson, J.D.: in *Harrison's Principles of Internal Medicine*, Isselbacher, K.J., Adams, R.D., Braunwald, E., Petersdorf, R.G., and Wilson, J.D. (eds.), 9th Edition, McGraw-Hill Book Company, New York City, l980, p. 1788.

II-6 CAUSES OF POLYURIA

I. Vasopressin deficiency (neurogenic diabetes insipidus)
  A. Acquired
    1. Idiopathic
    2. Trauma (accidental, surgical)
    3. Tumors (craniopharyngioma, metastasis)
    4. Granuloma (sarcoid, histiocytosis)
    5. Infectious (meningitis, encephalitis)
    6. Vascular (Sheehan's syndrome, aneurysms)
  B. Familial
II. Excessive water intake (primary polydipsia)
  A. Acquired
    1. Idiopathic
    2. Schizophrenia
III. Vasopressin insensitivity (nephrogenic diabetes insipidus)
  A. Acquired
    1. Infectious (pyelonephritis)
    2. Postobstructive (prostatic, ureteral)
    3. Vascular (sickle-cell disease, trait)
    4. Infiltrative (amyloid)
    5. Cystic (polycystic disease)
    6. Metabolic (hypokalemia, hypercalcemia)
    7. Granuloma (sarcoid)
    8. Toxic (lithium, demeclocycline, methoxyflurane)
    9. Solute overload (glucosuria, postobstructive)
  B. Familial

Adapted from: Robertson, G.L.: in *Endocrinology and Metabolism*, Felig, P., Baxter, J.D., Broadus, A.E., and Frohman, L.A. (eds.), 1st Edition, McGraw-Hill Book Company, New York, 1981, p. 262.

II-7 DIFFERENTIAL DIAGNOSIS OF THE SYNDROME OF INAPPROPRIATE ANTIDIURESIS (SIADH)

I. Tumors
  A. Bronchogenic carcinoma
  B. Carcinoma of duodenum
  C. Carcinoma of pancreas
  D. Thymoma
  E. Carcinoma of ureter
  F. Lymphoma
  G. Ewing's sarcoma
  H. Carcinoma of the prostate

II. Nonneoplastic diseases
   A. Trauma
   B. Pulmonary disease
       1. Pneumonia
       2. Cavitation (aspergillosis)
       3. Tuberculosis
       4. Positive-pressure breathing
       5. Lung abscess
   C. Central nervous system disorders
       1. Encephalitis or meningitis
       2. Head injury
       3. Brain abscess
       4. Encephalitis
       5. Guillain-Barré syndrome
       6. Subarachnoid hemorrhage or subdural hematoma
       7. Acute intermittent porphyria
       8. Peripheral neuropathy
       9. Psychosis
       10. Delirium tremens
       11. CSF leak
       12. Cerebrovascular accident
   D. SIADH in endocrine disease
       1. Addison's disease
       2. Myxedema
       3. Hypopituitarism
   E. "Idiopathic" SIADH
III. Drugs
   A. Vasopressin
   B. Oxytocin
   C. Vincristine
   D. Chlorpropamide
   E. Chlorothiazide, hydrochlorothiazide, hydroflumethiazide, and cyclothiazide
   F. Clofibrate
   G. Carbamazepine
   H. Nicotine
   I. Phenothiazines
   J. Cyclophosphamide
   K. Tricyclic antidepressants
   L. Narcotics

Adapted from: Robertson, G.L.: in *Endocrinology and Metabolism*, Felig, P., Baxter, J.D., Broadus, A.E., and Frohman, L.A. (eds.), 1st Edition, McGraw-Hill Book Company, New York, 1981, p. 269.

II-8 CAUSES OF HYPERTHYROIDISM

I. Grave's disease
II. Thyroiditis
   A. Subacute thyroiditis
   B. Painless thyroiditis
   C. Radiation thyroiditis
III. Exogenous hyperthyroidism
   A. Iatrogenic
   B. Factitious
   C. Iodine-induced
   D. Hashimoto's thyroiditis
   E. Silent thyroiditis
IV. Toxic multinodular goiter
V. Toxic uninodular goiter (thyroid adenoma)
VI. Ectopic hyperthyroidism (struma ovarii)
VII. Thyroid carcinoma
VIII. TSH excess
   A. Pituitary thyrotropin
   B. Trophoblastic tumors
   C. Pituitary insensitive to T_4 feedback inhibition

Adapted from: Spaulding, S.W., et al.: Frohman, L.A.: in *Endocrinology and Metabolism*, Felig, P., Baxter, J.D., Broadus, A.E., and Frohman, L.A. (eds.), 1st Edition, McGraw-Hill Book Company, New York, 1981, p. 303.

II-9 CLINICAL FEATURES OF HYPERTHYROIDISM

Symptoms	Physical signs	Diagnosis
Weight loss	Moist, warm, smooth skin	↑ T_4
Diarrhea	Tachycardia	↑ free T_4
Heat intolerance	Plummer's nails	↑ T_3
Nervousness	Ocular signs	↑ RAI uptake
Excessive sweating	Exophthalmos	↑ T_3 uptake
Emotional	Stare	
instability	Lid lag	
Polyphagia	Infrequent blinking	
Fatigue and	Difficulty with convergence	
weakness		
Palpitations	Thyromegaly	
	Thyroid bruit	
	Means-Lerman scratch/high	
	pitched pulmonic sound	
	Atrial arrhythmias (esp. atrial	
	fibrillation)	
	Heart failure	
	Hepatomegaly	
	Abnormal liver tests	
	Pretibial myxedema	

II-10 CAUSES OF HYPOTHYROIDISM

  I. Thyroidal hypothyroidism
    A. Insufficient functional tissue
      1. Primary atrophy
      2. Thyroiditis*
      3. Following ^{131}I therapy or thyroidectomy
      4. Thyroid dysgenesis
      5. Infiltrations*
    B. Defective biosynthesis
      1. Iodine deficiency*
      2. Congenital effects*
      3. Antithyroid agents*
      4. Iodine excess*
 II. Pituitary hypothyroidism
    A. Pituitary destruction
    B. Pituitary tumor
    C. Isolated TSH deficiency
III. Hypothalamic hypothyroidism
IV. Impaired peripheral sensitivity*

* Hypothyroidism may be accompanied by goiter in these cases.

Adapted from: Spaulding, S.W., et al.: in *Endocrinology and Metabolism*, Felig, P., Baxter, J.D., Broadus, A.E., and Frohman, L.A. (eds.), 1st Edition, McGraw-Hill Book Company, New York, 1981, p. 327.

II-11 CLASSIFICATION OF NONTOXIC GOITER

  I. Nontoxic diffuse goiter
    A. Endemic
      1. Iodine deficiency
      2. Iodine excess
      3. Dietary goitrogens
    B. Sporadic
      1. Congenital defect in thyroid hormone biosynthesis
      2. Chemical agents, e.g., lithium, thiocyanate, p-aminosalicylic acid
      3. Iodine deficiency
    C. Compensatory following subtotal thyroidectomy
 II. Nontoxic nodular goiter due to causes listed above
    A. Uninodular or multinodular
    B. Functional and/or nonfunctional

Modified from Werner SC: J Clin Endocrinol 29:860, 1969.

II-12 THYROID TUMOR

HISTOLOGICAL CLASSIFICATION OF EPITHELIAL THYROID TUMORS ACCORDING TO THE WORLD HEALTH ORGANIZATION

I. Epithelial tumors
   A. Benign
      1. Follicular adenoma
      2. Others
   B. Malignant
      1. Follicular carcinoma
      2. Papillary carcinoma
      3. Squamous cell carcinoma
      4. Undifferentiated (anaplastic) carcinoma
         a. Spindle cell type
         b. Giant cell type
         c. Small cell type
      5. Medullary carcinoma
II. Nonepithelial tumors
   A. Benign
   B. Malignant
      1. Fibrosarcoma
      2. Others
III. Miscellaneous tumors
   A. Carcinosarcoma
   B. Malignant hemangioendothelioma
   C. Malignant lymphoma
   D. Teratomas
IV. Secondary tumors

Histological Typing of Thyroid Tumors, International Histologic Classification of Tumors, no. 11, Geneva, World Health Organization, 1974.

CLINICAL STAGES OF THYROID CARCINOMA

Stage 1	Intrathyroidal lesions only
Stage 2	Nonfixed cervical metastases
Stage 3	Fixed lymph node metastases or invasion into the neck outside the thyroid
Stage 4	Thyroid tumors with metastatic disease outside the neck

Modified from: Smedal ML, Salzman FA, Meissner WA: Am J Roentgenol 99:352, 1967. Source adapted from: Burrow, G.N.: in *Endocrinology and Metabolism*, Felig, P., Baxter, J.D., Broadus, A.E., and Frohman, L.A. (eds.), 1st Edition, McGraw-Hill Book Company, New York, 1981, p. 371.

II-13 STATES ASSOCIATED WITH DECREASED PERIPHERAL CONVERSION OF T_4 TO T_3

I. Physiologic
  A. Fetal and early neonatal life
  B. Old age
II. Pathologic
  A. Fasting
  B. Malnutrition
  C. Systemic illness
  D. Physical trauma
  E. Postoperative state
  F. Drugs (propylthiouracil, dexamethasone, propranolol)
  G. Radiographic contrast agents (Oragrafin, Telepaque)

Ingbar, S.H., et al.: in *Harrison's Principles of Internal Medicine*, Issel-bacher, K.J., Adams, R.D., Braunwald, E., Petersdorf, R.G., and Wilson, J.D. (eds.), 9th Edition, McGraw-Hill Book Company, New York City, 1980, p. 1698.

II-14 ADRENAL CORTICAL INSUFFICIENCY

I. Etiology of primary adrenocortical insufficiency
   A. Idiopathic/autoimmune (≈80%)
   B. Tuberculosis (≈20%)
   C. Miscellaneous (≈1%)
      1. (1) Hemorrhage: sepsis, anticoagulants, coagulopathy, trauma, surgery, pregnancy, neonatal
         (2) Infarction: thrombosis, embolism, arteritis
      2. Fungal infection: histoplasmosis, coccidioidomycosis, blastomycosis, moniliasis, torulosis
      3. Metastatic
      4. Lymphoma
      5. Amyloidosis
      6. Sarcoidosis
      7. Hemochromatosis
      8. Surgery: bilateral adrenalectomy
      9. Enzyme inhibitors: metyrapone, aminoglutethimide, trilostane
      10. Cytotoxic agents: o,p'-DDD
      11. Congenital: adrenal hyperplasia, hypoplasia, familial glucocorticoid deficiency

Sources: Irvine WJ, Barnes EW: Adrenocortical insufficiency. Clin. Endocrinol. Metab. 1:549-594, 1972. Adapted from: Baxter, J.D., et al.: Frohman, L.A.: in *Endocrinology and MetabDH*Folism, Felig, P., Baxter, J.D., Broadus, A.E., and Frohman, L.A. (eds.), lst Edition, McGraw-Hill Book Company, New York, 1981, p. 448.

II. Clinical disorders associated with idiopathic adrenocortical insufficiency
   A. Primary ovarian failure
   B. Thyroid
      1. Thyrotoxicosis
      2. Hypothyroidism/chronic thyroiditis
   C. Diabetes mellitus
   D. Vitiligo
   E. Hypoparathyroidism
   F. Pernicious anemia
   G. Moniliasis

Sources: Irvine WJ, Barnes EW: Adrenocortical insufficiency. Clin. Endocrinol. Metab. 1:549-594, 1972. Adapted from: Baxter, J.D., et al.: in *Endocrinology and Metabolism*, Felig, P., Baxter, J.D., Broadus, A.E., and Frohman, L.A. (eds.), 1st Edition, McGraw-Hill Book Co pany, New York, 1981, p. 449.

II-15 CLINICAL FEATURES OF ADDISON'S DISEASE

Symptoms and physician signs
  I. Anorexia
  II. Weakness and easy fatigability
  III. Nausea and vomiting
  IV. Weight loss
  V. Salt craving
  VI. Diarrhea
  VII. Postural hypotension
  VIII. Hyperpigmentation
  IX. Personality changes
  X. Decrease in axillary and pubic hair

Diagnosis
  I. ↓ plasma cortisol
    A. Little increase after synthetic ACTH
    B. ↑ ACTH levels with primary adrenal failure
  II. ↓ urinary 17-hydroxy and 17-ketosteroid
  III. Hyponatremia
  IV. Hyperkalemia
  V. Anemia
  VI. Eosinophilia
  VII. Reduction in heart size

II-16 CUSHING'S SYNDROME
  I. Classification and Etiology

		Percent
A. ACTH dependent:		
	1. Cushing's disease	68
	2. Ectopic ACTH syndrome	15
B. ACTH independent:		
	1. Adrenal adenoma	9
	2. Adrenal carcinoma	8
		100

Huff TA: Clinical syndromes related to disorders of adrenocorticotrophic hormone, In Allen MB, Makesh VB (eds). The Pituitary: A Current Review. New York, Academic Press, 1977. pp. 153-168.

  II. Tumors Most Frequently Causing the Ectopic ACTH Syndrome
    A. Oat cell carcinoma of the lung
    B. Thymoma
    C. Pancreatic islet cell carcinoma
    D. Carcinoid tumors (lung, gut, pancreas, ovary)
    E. Thyroid medullary carcinoma
    F. Pheochromocytoma and related tumors

Adapted from: Baxter, J.D., et al.: in Frohman, L.A.: in *Endocrinology and Metabolism*, Felig, P., Baxter, J.D., Broadus, A.E., and Frohman, L.A. (eds.), 1st Edition, McGraw-Hill Book Company, New York, 1981, p. 469.

II-17 CLINICAL FEATURES OF CUSHING'S SYNDROME

Clinical features

I. Typical facial features and habitus
II. Weight gain
III. Weakness and easy fatigability
IV. Amenorrhea
V. Personality changes
VI. Polyuria, polydipsia
VII. Hypertension
VIII. Hirsutism, striae, ecchymosis
IX. Edema
X. Clitoral hypertrophy

Diagnosis

I. Plasma cortisol usually ↑
   A. No suppression with pm dexamethasone
II. ↑ urinary 17 hydroxycorticoid
III. Suppression of plasma cortisol and urinary hydroxycorticoids by low or high dose dexamethasone
IV. Mild leukocytosis
V. Eosinopenia
VI. Hypokalemic alkalosis
VII. Hyperglycemia
VIII. CT scan may be of value

II-18 SYNDROME OF PRIMARY ALDOSTERONISM

I. Etiology
   A. Aldosterone-producing adenoma
   B. Adrenocortical hyperplasia
      1. Idiopathic aldosteronism (aldosterone production-nonsuppressible)
      2. Indeterminate aldosteronism (aldosterone production-suppressible)
      3. Glucocorticoid-suppressible aldosteronism
      4. Surgically remediable aldosteronism (?)
   C. Adrenocortical carcinoma
II. Clinical features
   A. Symptoms and signs
      1. Hypertension
      2. Muscle weakness
      3. Polyuria
      4. Polydipsia
   B. Diagnosis
      1. Hypokalemia
      2. Hypernatremia (occasional)
      3. Alkaline to neutral urine pH
      4. Metabolic alkalosis
      5. Hyperglycemia
      6. Failure of plasma renin to rise normally
         a. diuretics
         b. upright
         c. sodium depletion
      7. CT scan may be helpful

II-19 CLASSIFICATION OF SECONDARY HYPERALDOSTERONISM

Primary abnormality	Potassium loss	Edema	Hypertension	Effect of sodium load
Extrarenal sodium loss Hemorrhage Thermal stress Gastrointestinal loss	Absent	Absent	Absent	Repairs deficit
Sodium restriction	Absent	Absent	Absent	Repairs deficit
Abnormal distribution of sodium excess Congestive heart failure Nephrotic syndrome Cirrhosis with ascites Idiopathic edema	Present	Present	Absent	Worsens edema
Abnormal renal electrolyte loss Salt-losing renal disease* Bartter's syndrome Diuretic abuse Renal tubular acidosis	Present	Absent	Absent	Variable
Other renal lesions Renal artery stenosis Unilateral renal ischemia Accelerated hypertension Renin-secreting tumor Chronic renal failure*	Present (except*)	Absent	Present	May worsen hypertension
Excessive potassium intake	Present	Absent	Absent	May facilitate kaluresis
Luteal phase of menstrual cycle and pregnancy	Absent	May be present	Usually present	Suppresses renin and aldosterone

Modified from Stockigt JR: Mineralocorticoid excess, In James VHT (ed.): The Adrenal Gland. New York, Raven Press, 1979, pp. 197-242.

Adapted from: Baxter, J.D., et al.: in *Endocrinology and Metabolism*, Felig, P., Baxter, J.D., Broadus, A.E., and Frohman, L.A. (eds.), 1st Edition, McGraw-Hill Book Company, New York, 1981, p. 485.

II-20   CAUSES OF HYPOMAGNESEMIA AND MAGNESIUM DEPLETION

I. Decreased intake and/or absorption
   A. Protein-calorie malnutrition
   B. Losses of gastrointestinal fluids
   C. Malabsorption
   D. Primary hypomagnesemia
II. Renal losses
   A. Nonazotemic tubular dysfunction
   B. Diuretics
   C. Primary and secondary aldosteronism
   D. Idiopathic hypomagnesemia
III. Magnesium depletion and miscellaneous disorders
   A. Chronic alcoholism
   B. Diabetic ketoacidosis
   C. Bone resorption
   D. Hyperthyroidism

Adapted from: Broadus, A.E.: Frohman, L.A.: in *Endocrinology and Metabolism*, Felig, P., Baxter, J.D., Broadus, A.E., and Frohman, L.A. (eds.), 1st Edition, McGraw-Hill Book Company, New York, 1981, p. 1070.

II-21 CLASSIFICATION OF DIABETES MELLITUS

I. Spontaneous diabetes mellitus
   A. Type I or insulin-dependent diabetes (formerly called juvenile-onset diabetes)
   B. Type II or insulin-independent diabetes (formerly called maturity-onset diabetes)
II. Secondary diabetes
   A. Pancreatic disease (pancreoprivic diabetes, e.g., pancreatectomy, pancreatic insufficiency, hemochromatosis)
   B. Hormonal: excess secretion of contrainsulin hormones (e.g., acromegaly, Cushing's syndrome, pheochromocytoma)
   C. Drug induced (e.g., potassium-losing diuretics, contra- insulin hormones, psychoactive agents, diphenylhydantoin)
   D. Associated with complex genetic syndromes (e.g., ataxia telangiectasia, Laurence-Moon-Biedl syndrome, myotonic dystrophy, Friedreich's ataxia)
III. Impaired glucose tolerance (formerly called chemical diabetes, asymptomatic diabetes, latent diabetes, and subclinical diabetes): normal fasting plasma glucose, and 2-h value on glucose tolerance test >140 mg/dL but <200 mg/dL.
IV. Gestational diabetes: glucose intolerance which has its onset in pregnancy

---

Sources: National Diabetes Data Group: Diabetes 28:1039, 1979. Adapted from: Felig, P.: Frohman, L.A.: in *Endocrinology and Metabolism*, Felig, P., Baxter, J.D., Broadus, A.E., and Frohman, L.A. (eds.), 1st Edition, McGraw-Hill Book Company, New York, 1981, p. 799.

II-22 PRECIPITATING FACTORS IN DIABETIC KETOACIDOSIS

I. Infection
   A. Urinary tract
   B. Pneumonias
   C. Cellulitis
   D. Periodontal
   E. Central nervous system
   F. Septicemia
II. Metabolic/Endocrine
   A. Uremia
   B. Hypothyroidism
   C. Cushing's syndrome
III. Dietary indiscretion
IV. Not taking insulin
V. Pregnancy
VI. Myocardial infarction
VII. CVA
VIII. Drugs
   A. Thiazides
   B. Corticosteroids
IX. Acute pancreatitis

II-23 MAJOR CAUSES OF FASTING HYPOGLYCEMIA

I. Conditions primarily due to underproduction of glucose
   A. Hormone deficiencies
      1. Hypopituitarism
      2. Adrenal insufficiency
      3. Catecholamine deficiency
      4. Glucagon deficiency
   B. Enzyme defects
      1. Glucose 6-phosphatase
      2. Liver phosphorylase
      3. Pyruvate carboxylase
      4. Phosphoenolpyruvate carboxykinase
      5. Fructose I,6-diphosphatase
      6. Glycogen synthetase
   C. Substrate deficiency
      1. Ketotic hypoglycemia of infancy
      2. Severe malnutrition, muscle wasting(?)
      3. Late pregnancy (?)
   D. Acquired liver disease
      1. Hepatic congestion
      2. Severe hepatitis
      3. Cirrhosis
   E. Drugs
      1. Alcohol
      2. Propranolol
      3. Salicylates
II. Conditions primarily due to overutilization of glucose
   A. Hyperinsulinism
      1. Insulinoma
      2. Exogenous insulin
      3. Sulfonylureas
      4. Immune disease with insulin antibodies
   B. Appropriate insulin levels
      1. Extrapancreatic tumors
      2. Carnitine deficiency
      3. Cachexia with fat depletion

Adapted from: Foster, D.W., and Rubenstein, A.H.: in *Harrison's Principles of Internal Medicine*, Isselbacher, K.J., Adams, R.D., Braunwald, E., Petersdorf, R.G., and Wilson, J.D. (eds.), 9th Edition, McGraw-Hill Book Company, New York City, 1980, p. 1759.

II-24 INSULIN RESISTANT STATES

I. Insulin resistance without acanthosis nigricans
  A. Obesity
  B. Insulin antibodies
  C. Werner's syndrome
II. Insulin resistance with acanthosis nigricans
  A. Due to receptor abnormality
    1. Receptor deficiency
    2. Antibody to insulin receptor
  B. Lipodystrophic states
  C. Ataxia telangiectasia
  D. Alström's syndrome
  E. Syndrome of familial insulin resistance

Adapted from: Foster, D.W.: in *Harrison's Principles of Internal Medicine*, Isselbacher, K.J., Adams, R.D., Braunwald, E., Petersdorf, R.G., and Wilson, J.D. (eds.), 9th Edition, McGraw-Hill Book Company, New York City, 1980, p. 1753.

II-25 A CLASSIFICATION OF THE OBESITIES

I. Etiologic
   A. Hypothalamic dysfunction
      1. Tumors
      2. Inflammation
      3. Trauma and surgical injury
      4. Increased intracranial pressure
      5. Functional changes causing hyperinsulinemia?
   B. Endocrine
      1. Glucocorticoid excess: Cushing's syndrome
      2. Thyroid hormone deficiency: hypothyroidism
      3. Hypopituitarism
      4. Gonadal deficiency: primary and secondary hypogonadism
      5. Hyperinsulinism: insulinoma, excess exogenous insulin
   C. Genetic
      1. Inherited predisposition to obesity
      2. Genetic syndromes associated with obesity:
         a. Prader-Willi syndrome
         b. Alström's syndrome
         c. Laurence-Moon-Bardet-Biedl syndrome
         d. Morgagni-Morel syndrome: hyperostosis frontalis interna
         e. Down's syndrome?
         f. Pseudo- and pseudopseudohypoparathyroidism?
   D. Nutritional
      1. Maternal nutritional factors?
      2. Infant feeding practices?
   E. Drugs
      1. Phenothiazines
      2. Insulin
      3. Corticosteroids
      4. Cyproheptidine
      5. Tricyclic antidepressants
II. Anatomic
   A. Hypercellular-hypertrophic: early age of onset, severe obesity
   B. Hypertrophic-normal cellular: adult onset, milder obesity
III. Contributory factors
   A. Familial influences
   B. Physical inactivity
   C. Dietary factors: eating patterns, type of diet
   D. Socioeconomic
   E. Educational
   F. Cultural-ethnic
   G. Psychologic

Adapted from: Salans, L.B.: in *Endocrinology and Metabolism*, Felig, P., Baxter, J.D., Broadus, A.E., and Frohman, L.A. (eds.), 1st Edition, Mc-Graw-Hill Book Company, New York, 1981, p. 904.

II-26 HYPERCALCEMIC CONDITIONS ARRANGED BY CATEGORY IN DESCENDING ORDER OF APPROXIMATE FREQUENCY

I. Primary hyperparathyroidism
   A. Sporadic
   B. Clinical variants and familial syndromes
II. Neoplastic diseases
   A. Local osteolysis
   B. Humoral hypercalcemia of malignancy (PTH)
   C. Other factors: prostaglandins, vitamin D-like sterols
III. Endocrinopathies
   A. Thyrotoxicosis
   B. Adrenal insufficiency
   C. Pheochromocytoma
IV. Medications
   A. Thiazide diuretics
   B. Vitamins A and D
   C. Milk-alkali syndrome
   D. Lithium
V. Sarcoidosis and other granulomatous diseases
VI. Miscellaneous conditions
   A. Immobilization
   B. Acute renal failure
   C. Idiopathic hypercalcemia of infancy

Adapted from: Broadus, A.E.: in *Endocrinology and Metabolism*, Felig, P., Baxter, J.D., Broadus, A.E., and Frohman, L.A. (eds.), 1st Edition, McGraw-Hill Book Company, New York, 1981, p. 1019.

II-27 HYPOPARATHYROIDISM

I. Postoperative hypocalcemia and hypoparathyroidism
II. Idiopathic hypoparathyroidism
   A. Isolated
   B. Associated with atrophic polyendocrine failure
III. Other acquired forms of functional hypoparathyroidism
   A. Nonsurgical parathyroid damage
   B. Parathyroid infiltration
   C. Hypomagnesemia
IV. Pseudohypoparathyroidism
V. Neonatal hypocalcemic syndromes
   A. Early and late neonatal hypocalcemia
   B. Secondary hypoparathyroidism
   C. DiGeorge syndrome and idiopathic hypoparathyroidism

Adapted from: Broadus, A.E.: in *Endocrinology and Metabolism*, Felig, P., Baxter, J.D., Broadus, A.E., and Frohman, L.A. (eds.), 1st Edition, McGraw-Hill Book Company, New York, 1981, p. 1054.

II-28 NONHYPOPARATHYROID HYPOCALCEMIA CONDITIONS

   I. Renal insufficiency
  II. Vitamin D deficiency, rickets, and osteomalacia
     A. Simple vitamin D deficiency
     B. Intestinal malabsorption
     C. Hepatic and biliary disorders
     D. Anticonvulsant therapy
     E. Vitamin D-dependent rickets
     F. Vitamin D-resistant (hypophosphatemic) rickets and osteomalacia
       1. Familial
       2. Sporadic
       3. Tumor-associated
     G. Fanconi syndromes
     H. Distal renal tubular acidosis
 III. Acute pancreatitis
 IV. Malignancy
     A. Osteoblastic metastases
     B. Rapid tumor lysis
  V. Medications
     A. Mithramycin
     B. Citrated blood
     C. Fluoride intoxication
 VI. Hungry bone syndrome

Adapted from: Broadus, A.E., Frohman, L.A.: in *Endocrinology and Metabolism*, Felig, P., Baxter, J.D., Broadus, A.E., and Frohman, L.A. (eds.), 1st Edition, McGraw-Hill Book Company, New York, 1981, p. 1063.

II-29 CLASSIFICATION OF OSTEOMALACIA AND RICKETS

I. Reduction of circulating vitamin D metabolites
  A. Inadequate ultraviolet light exposure and inadequate dietary vitamin D
  B. Vitamin D malabsorption
     1. Small intestinal disease
     2. Pancreatic insufficiency
     3. Insufficient bile salts
  C. Abnormal vitamin D metabolism
     1. Liver disease
     2. Chronic renal failure
     3. Systemic acidosis
     4. Drugs (anticonvulsants, glutethimide)
     5. Mesenchymal tumors, prostatic cancer
     6. Vitamin D-dependent rickets (25-hydroxyvitamin D-lα-hydroxylase deficiency)
  D. Renal loss
     l. Nephrotic syndrome
II. Peripheral resistance to vitamin D
  A. Vitamin D-dependent rickets, type II
  B. Anticonvulsant drugs
  C. Chronic renal failure
III. Hypophosphatemia
  A. Renal phosphate wasting
     1. Hypophosphatemic rickets
        a. Familial X-linked
        b. Autosomal recessive
        c. Sporadic
     2. Hypophosphatemic osteomalacia
        a. Familial X-linked
        b. Sporadic
     3. Fanconi syndrome
     4. Mesenchymal tumors, fibrous dysplasias, epidermal nevus syndrome, prostatic cancer
     5. Primary hyperparathyroidism
  B. Malnutrition
  C. Malabsorption due to gastrointestinal disease or phosphate-binding antacids
  D. Chronic dialysis
IV. Miscellaneous
  A. Inhibitors of calcification
     1. Sodium fluoride
     2. Disodium etidronate
  B. Calcium deficiency
  C. Hypophosphatasia
  D. Fibrogenesis imperfecta ossium

Adapted from: Singer, F.R.: Frohman, L.A.: in *Endocrinology and Metabolism*, Felig, P., Baxter, J.D., Broadus, A.E., and Frohman, L.A. (eds.), 1st Edition, McGraw-Hill Book Company, New York, 1981, p. 1088.

II-30 CLASSIFICATION OF OSTEOPOROSIS

I. Senile
II. Endocrine abnormality
   A. Estrogen deficiency
   B. Testosterone deficiency
   C. Cushing's syndrome
   D. Thyrotoxicosis
   E. Primary hyperparathyroidism
   F. Diabetes mellitus
III. Nutritional abnormality
   A. Vitamin C deficiency
   B. Protein deficiency
IV. Immobilization or weightlessness
V. Hematologic malignancy
   A. Multiple myeloma
   B. Leukemia
   C. Lymphoma
VI. Genetic
   A. Osteogenesis imperfecta
   B. Ehlers-Danlos syndrome
   C. Homocystinuria
   D. Marfan's syndrome
   E. Menkes' syndrome
VII. Systemic mastocytosis
VIII. Heparin therapy
IX. Rheumatoid arthritis
X. Chronic liver disease
XI. Juvenile osteoporosis
XII. Idiopathic

Adapted from: Singer, F.R.: Frohman, L.A.: in *Endocrinology and Metabolism*, Felig, P., Baxter, J.D., Broadus, A.E., and Frohman, L.A. (eds.), lst Edition, McGraw-Hill Book Company, New York, 1981, p. 1096.

II-31 CLINICAL RISK FACTORS FOR CALCIUM STONE FORMATION

    I. Positive family history
   II. Dehydration
  III. Medications
      A. Vitamins A, D, and C
      B. Absorbable antacids
      C. Acetazolamide
  IV. Urine pH
   V. Diet
  VI. Hypercalciuria
 VII. Hyperoxaluria
VIII. Hyperuricosuria

Adapted from: Broadus, A.E.: Frohman, L.A.: in *Endocrinology and Metabolism*, Felig, P., Baxter, J.D., Broadus, A.E., and Frohman, L.A. (eds.), 1st Edition, McGraw-Hill Book Company, New York, 1981, p. 1145.

II-32 CAUSES OF HIRSUTISM IN FEMALES

    I. Familial
   II. Idiopathic
  III. Ovarian
      A. Polycystic ovaries; hilus-cell hyperplasia
      B. Tumor; arrhenoblastoma, hilus cell, adrenal rest
  IV. Adrenal
      A. Congenital adrenal hyperplasia
      B. Noncongenital adrenal hyperplasia (Cushing's)
      C. Tumor: virilizing carcinoma or adenoma
   V. Drugs: minoxidil, androgens

Adapted from: Williams, G.W., Dluny, R.G., Thorn, G.W.: in *Harrison's Principles of Internal Medicine*, Isselbacher, K.J., Adams, R.D., Braunwald, E., Petersdorf, R.G., and Wilson, J.D. (eds.), 9th Edition, McGraw-Hill Book Company, New York City, 1980, p. 1728.

II-33 CLASSIFICATION OF THE ENDOCRINE DISORDERS OF THE OVARY

I. Ovarian hypofunction
   A. Primary
      1. General
         a. Gonadal dysgenesis (Turner syndrome and its variants)
         b. Autoimmune disorders with anti-steroid- producing cell antibodies
         c. 17 alpha-hydroxylase deficiency
         d. Iatrogenic (pelvic irradiation, cytotoxic drugs)
         e. "Resistant ovary" syndrome
         f. Menopause, premature and physiological
   B. Secondary
      1. General
         a. Hypothalamic disorders
         b. Hypopituitarism
         c. Constitutional and metabolic disturbances
      2. Compartmental
         a. Anovulatory bleeding
         b. Inadequate luteal phase
II. Ovarian hyperfunction
   A. Primary
      1. Feminizing tumors
      2. Masculinizing tumors
   B. Secondary
      1. General: true precocious puberty
      2. Compartmental
         a. Persistent follicle cyst
         b. Corpus luteum cyst
         c. Stein-Leventhal syndrome and hyperthecosis
III. Ovarian dysfunction
   A. Choriocarcinoma
   B. Struma ovarii
   C. Carcinoid

Adapted from: McArthur, J.W.: in *Harrison's Principles of Internal Medicine*, Isselbacher, K.J., Adams, R.D., Braunwald, E., Petersdorf, R.G., and Wilson, J.D. (eds.), 9th Edition, McGraw-Hill Book Company, New York City, 1980, p. 1781.

II-34 DIFFERENTIAL DIAGNOSIS OF GYNECOMASTIA

I. Physiological gynecomastia
  A. Newborn
  B. Adolescence
  C. Aging
II. Pathological gynecomastia
  A. Deficient production or action of testosterone
    1. Congenital anorchia
    2. Klinefelter syndrome
    3. Androgen resistance (testicular feminization and Reifenstein syndrome)
    4. Defects in testosterone synthesis
    5. Secondary testicular failure (viral orchitis, trauma castration, neurological and granulomatous diseases, renal failure)
  B. Increased estrogen production
    1. Estrogen secretion
      a. True hermaphroditism
      b. Testicular tumors
      c. Carcinoma of the lung
    2. Increased substrate for peripheral aromatase
      a. Adrenal disease
      b. Liver disease
      c. Starvation
      d. Thyrotoxicosis
    3. Increase in peripheral aromatase
  C. Drugs
    1. Inhibitors of testosterone synthesis and/or action (spironolactone, cimetidine)
    2. Estrogens (diethylstilbestrol, birth control pills, digitalis, marijuana, heroin)
    3. Gonadotropins
    4. Unknown mechanisms (busulphan, ethionamide, isoniazid, methyldopa, tricyclic antidepressants)

Adapted from: Emerson, K., Wilson, J.D.: in *Harrison's Principles of Internal Medicine*, Isselbacher, K.J., Adams, R.D., Braunwald, E., Petersdorf, R.G., and Wilson, J.D. (eds.), 9th Edition, McGraw-Hill Book Company, New York City, 1980, p. 1789.

II-35 HYPERLIPIDEMIC DISORDERS

I. Exogenous hyperlipemia (chylomicrons)
  A. Familial lipoprotein lipase deficiency
  B. C-II apolipoprotein deficiency
  C. Secondary disorders
    1. Dysglobulinemias
    2. S.L.E.

54

II. Endogenous hyperlipemia (VLDL)
   A. Familial hypertriglyceridemia (mild form)
   B. Familial multiple lipoprotein-type hyperlipidemia
   C. Sporadic hypertriglyceridemia
   D. Tangier disease
   E. Secondary disorders
      1. Diabetic hyperlipemia
      2. Uremia
      3. Nephrotic syndrome
      4. Dysglobulinemias
      5. Lipodystrophies
      6. Hypopituitarism
III. Mixed hyperlipemia (VLDL + chylomicrons)
   A. Familial hypertriglyceridemia (severe form)
   B. Familial lipoprotein lipase deficiency (during pregnancy)
   C. Secondary disorders (same as
      II. E. above)
IV. Hypercholesterolemia (LDL)
   A. Familial hypercholesterolemia (LDL receptor defects)
   B. Familial multiple lipoprotein-type hyperlipidemia
   C. Polygenic hypercholesterolemia
   D. Secondary disorders
      1. Nephrotic syndrome
      2. Hypothyroidism
      3. Dysglobulinemias
      4. Cushing's syndrome
      5. Hepatoma
      6. Acute intermittent porphyria
V. Combined hyperlipidemia (LDL + VLDL)
   A. Familial multiple lipoprotein-type hyperlipidemia
   B. Unclassified
   C. Secondary disorders
      1. Nephrotic syndrome
      2. Hypothyroidism
      3. Dysglobulinemias
      4. Cushing's syndrome
      5. Glucocorticoid use
VI. Remnant hyperlipidemia (Beta-VLDL)
   A. Familial dysbetalipoproteinemia
   B. Unclassified
   C. Secondary disorders
      1. Hypothyroidism
      2. Systemic lupus erythematosis

Modified from: Havel, R.J., Goldstein, J.L., and Brown, M.S.: In Bondy, PK, and Rosenberg, LE (eds.): Metabolic Control and Disease. 8th ed., 1980, Philadelphia, W.B. Saunders Company, p. 412.

III—Gastroenterology

III-1 CLASSIFICATION OF ESOPHAGEAL MOTILITY DISORDERS

I. Primary
  A. Achalasia
  B. Diffuse esophageal spasm
  C. Variants of achalasia and diffuse esophageal spasm
II. Secondary
  A. Collagen disease
    1. Scleroderma
    2. Systemic lupus erythematosus
    3. Raynaud's disease
    4. Dermatomyositis, polymyositis
  B. Physical, chemical and pharmacologic
    1. Vagotomy
    2. Radiation
    3. Chemical: reflux esophagitis
    4. Drugs (atropine, belladonna alkaloids)
  C. Neurologic disease
    1. Cerebrovascular disease
    2. Pseudobulbar palsy
    3. Multiple sclerosis
    4. Amyotrophic lateral sclerosis
    5. Bulbar poliomyelitis
    6. Parkinsonism
  D. Muscle disease
    1. Myotonic dystrophy
    2. Muscular dystrophy
    3. Myasthenia gravis (motor end-plate)
  E. Infection
    1. Chagas' disease (Trypanosoma cruzi)
    2. Diphtheria
    3. Tetanus
  F. Metabolic
    1. Diabetes
    2. Alcoholism
    3. Thyrotoxicosis
    4. Myxedema
  G. Miscellaneous
    1. Idiopathic intestinal pseudo-obstruction
    2. Amyloidosis

Greenberger, N.J.: *Gastrointestinal Disorders: A Pathophysiological Approach*, 2nd Edition, Year Book Medical Publishers, Chicago, 1981, p. 32.

III-2 ACHALASIA

I. Pathophysiology
  A. Denervation: neuropathology of achalasia
    1. Absence or degeneration of esophageal myenteric ganglion cells
    2. Vagus nerve electron-microscopic alterations: break in continuity of axon-Schwann membranes; swelling of axons; fragmentation of neurofilaments; mitochondrial degeneration in axoplasma
    3. Vagal nucleus: decrease in dorsal motor cells; cytologic distortion of remaining cells
  B. Functional neuropharmacology
    1. Excessive motor response of the distal esophagus to cholinergic drugs
    2. Supersensitivity of lower esophageal sphincter to gastrin; gastric acidification produces reduction in elevated lower esophageal tone to baseline
    3. Other factors: emotional stress, heredity
II. Clinical Features
  A. Symptoms: dysphagia for liquids and solids; odynophagia occasionally; regurgitation; tracheobronchial aspiration with pulmonary changes
  B. Signs: weight loss; halitosis; occasionally signs of pulmonary inflammation
III. Diagnosis
  A. Radiography: esophageal dilatation; distal esophagus terminates in a "beak"; aperistalsis; stasis
  B. Esophageal manometry: upper sphincter normal; aperistalsis in body of esophagus; failure of lower esophagus sphincter to relax completely; elevated lower esophageal sphincter resting pressure; hypersensitivity of lower esophageal sphincter to cholinergic drugs
  C. Esophagoscopy: exclude carcinoma, benign stricture; esophageal dilatation; esophagitis
IV. Treatment
  A. Brusque dilatation: forceful dilatation of inferior sphincter with pneumatic or hydrostatic balloon dilator; satisfactory results in 60-75%
  B. Surgical therapy: distal esophageal myotomy; satisfactory results 80%

Greenberger, N.J.: *Gastrointestinal Disorders: A Pathophysiological Approach*, 2nd Edition, Year Book Medical Publishers, Chicago, 1981, p. 33.

III-3 CONDITIONS ASSOCIATED WITH HYPERGASTRINEMIA AND DIAGNOSIS OF ZOLLINGER-ELLISON SYNDROME (ZES)

I. Conditions associated with hypergastrinemia
   A. With acid hypersecretion
      1. Gastrinoma (ZES)
      2. Antral G cell hyperplasia
      3. Isolated retained gastric antrum
      4. Massive small intestinal resection
      5. Hyperparathyroidism
      6. Pyloric outlet obstruction
   B. With variable acid secretion
      1. Hyperthyroidism
      2. Chronic renal failure
      3. Pheochromocytoma
   C. With acid hyposecretion
      1. Pernicious anemia
      2. Atrophic gastritis
      3. Gastric carcinoma
      4. After vagotomy and pyloroplasty

II. Serum gastrin levels in ZES
   A. >1000 pg/ml with $\uparrow$ [H$^+$] secretion—virtually diagnostic of ZES
   B. 500-1000 pg/ml—strongly suggestive of ZES
   C. 200-500 pg/ml—equivocal; 40% of patients with ZES have a gastrin level in this range

III. Provocative test for ZES
   A. Secretin injection (2 units/kg/I.V.) $\rightarrow$ $\uparrow$ in serum gastrin > 200 pg/ml (positive in 90-95% of ZES patients)

Greenberger, N.J.: *Gastrointestinal Disorders: A Pathophysiologic Approach*. 2nd Edition, Year Book Medical Publishers, Chicago, 1981, p. 97.

III-4 ATROPHIC GASTRITIS

Features	Type A	Type B
Involvement	Body and fundus	Antrum only
Serum gastrin	+	−
Parietal cell antibody	+	−
Antibodies to gastrin-producing cells	−	+
Pernicious anemia	+	−
Intrinsic factor antibodies	+	−
Autoimmune systemic disorders	+	−
Diabetes mellitus*		
Thyroid disease*		
Hashimoto's thyroiditis		
Myxedema		
Adrenal insufficiency		

Modified from Vandeli, C., et al.: N. Engl. J. Med. 300:1406, 1979.
(+) = present; (−) = absent.
*Frequently present in patients with Type A.

III-5 DELAYED GASTRIC EMPTYING

I. Gastric retention due to pyloric outlet obstruction
   A. Chronic duodenal ulcer diseases
   B. Idiopathic hypertrophic pyloric stenosis
   C. Crohn's disease of the stomach and/or duodenum
   D. Eosinophilic gastroenteritis
   E. Carcinoma of the stomach
   F. Carcinoma of the duodenum or pancreas
II. Acute gastric retention due to mechanical obstruction
   A. Pain
      1. Renal colic
      2. Biliary colic
      3. Recent surgery
   B. Trauma
      1. Retroperitoneal hematoma
      2. Ruptured spleen
      3. Urinary tract injury
   C. Inflammation and infection
      1. Pancreatitis
      2. Peritonitis
      3. Appendicitis
      4. Sepsis
      5. Acute viral gastroenteritis
   D. Immobilization
      1. Body plaster casts
      2. Paraplegia
      3. Postoperative states
   E. Acute gastric retention due to metabolic and electrolyte abnormalities
      1. Diabetic ketoacidosis
      2. Alcoholic ketoacidosis
      3. Myxedema
      4. Acute porphyria
      5. Hepatic coma
      6. Hypokalemia
      7. Hypocalcemia
      8. Hypercalcemia
III. Chronic gastric retention
   A. Neural and smooth muscle disorders
      1. Bulbar poliomyelitis
      2. Brain tumor
      3. Demyelinating diseases (multiple sclerosis)
      4. Vagotomy usually with prior gastric surgery
      5. Scleroderma
      6. Idiopathic intestinal pseudo-obstruction

III-5 DELAYED GASTRIC EMPTYING

B. Metabolic disorders
   1. Diabetes mellitus (vagal neuropathy may be present)
   2. Myxedema
   3. Drugs
      a. Anticholinergics
      b. Opiates (morphine, codeine, etc.)
      c. Ganglionic blockers
      d. Aluminum-containing antacids
      e. Pectin and ?psyllium hydrophilic mucilloids
   4. Psychiatric disease
      a. Anorexia nervosa
   5. Idiopathic
      a. Antecedent viral illnesses

Greenberger, N.J.: *Gastrointestinal Disorders: A Pathophysiological Approach*, 2nd Edition, Year Book Medical Publishers, Chicago, 1981, p. 110.

III-6 DIAGNOSIS OF ANOREXIA NERVOSA*

I. Age of onset before 25 yr
II. Anorexia with weight loss ≥ 25% of original body weight
III. Distorted, implacable attitude toward eating, food, or weight that overrides hunger, admonitions, reassurance, and threats, e.g.:
   A. Denial of illness with failure to recognize nutritional needs
   B. Enjoyment in losing weight
   C. Desired body image of extreme thinness with evidence that it is rewarding to achieve and maintain this state
   D. Unusual hoarding or handling of food
IV. No known medical illness to account for anorexia and weight loss
V. No other psychiatric disorder
VI. At least two of the following:
   A. Amenorrhea
   B. Lanugo
   C. Bradycardia
   D. Overactivity
   E. Bulimia
   F. Vomiting (may be self-induced)

*From Gastroenterology 77:1117, 1979.

III-7 CLASSIFICATION OF THE MALABSORPTION SYNDROMES

I. Inadequate digestion
   A. Postgastrectomy steatorrhea†
   B. Deficiency or inactivation of pancreatic lipase
      1. Exocrine pancreatic insufficiency
         a. Chronic pancreatitis
         b. Pancreatic carcinoma
         c. Cystic fibrosis
         d. Pancreatic resection
      2. Ulcerogenic tumor of the pancreas (Zollinger-Ellison syndrome†)
II. Reduced intestinal bile salt concentration (with impaired formation of micellar lipid)
   A. Liver disease
      1. Parenchymal liver disease
      2. Cholestasis (intrahepatic or extrahepatic)
   B. Abnormal bacterial proliferation in the small bowel
      1. Afferent loop stasis
      2. Strictures
      3. Fistulas
      4. Blind loops
      5. Multiple diverticula of the small bowel
      6. Hypomotility states (diabetes, scleroderma); intestinal pseudo-obstruction
   C. Interrupted enterohepatic circulation of bile salts
      1. Ileal resection
      2. Ileal inflammatory disease (regional ileitis)
   D. Drug-induced (by sequestration or precipitation of bile salts)
      1. Neomycin
      2. Calcium carbonate
      3. Cholestyramine
III. Inadequate absorptive surface
   A. Intestinal resection or bypass
      1. Mesenteric vascular disease with massive intestinal resection
      2. Regional enteritis with multiple bowel resection
      3. Jejunoileal bypass
   B. Gastroileostomy
IV. Lymphatic obstruction
   A. Intestinal lymphangiectasia
   B. Whipple's disease†
   C. Lymphoma†
   D. Kohlmeier-Degos (primary progressive arterial occlusive disease)†

III-7 CLASSIFICATION OF THE MALABSORPTION SYNDROMES (CONTINUED)

   V. Cardiovascular disorders
- A. Constrictive pericarditis
- B. Congestive heart failure
- C. Mesenteric vascular insufficiency
- D. Collagen vascular disease with vasculitis

  VI. Endocrine and metabolic disorders
- A. Diabetes mellitus
- B. Hypoparathyroidism
- C. Adrenal insufficiency
- D. Hyperthyroidism
- E. Ulcerogenic tumor of the pancreas (Zollinger-Ellison syndrome†)
- F. Carcinoid syndrome

 VII. Primary mucosal absorptive defects
- A. Inflammatory or infiltrate disorders
  1. Regional enteritis†
  2. Amyloidosis
  3. Scleroderma†
  4. Lymphoma†
  5. Eosinophilic enteritis
  6. Tropical sprue
  7. Infectious enteritis (e.g., salmonellosis)
  8. Mucosal lesions associated with intestinal bacterial growth†
- B. Biochemical or genetic abnormalities
  1. Celiac sprue
  2. Abetalipoproteinemia
  3. Hartnup disease
  4. Cystinuria
  5. Hypogammaglobulinemia

† = multiple mechanisms responsible for malabsorption

III-8 CELIAC SPRUE

DIAGNOSIS OF CELIAC SPRUE

I. Evidence of malabsorption
  A. Isolated or generalized
     1. ↓ D-xylose, steatorrhea, ↓ Ca#, Fe#, albumin, cholesterol, carotenes, B_{12} absorption, ↑ protime, etc.
II. Abnormal small bowel mucosal biopsy
III. Improvement (clinical, laboratory tests, intestinal histology) with gluten-free diet
IV. Exacerbation of symptoms, diarrhea, and steatorrhea with gluten challenge
  A. Should be used only in equivocal cases

FAILURE TO RESPOND TO GLUTEN-FREE DIET

I. Incorrect diagnosis
II. Nonadherence to gluten-free diet
III. Unsuspected concurrent disease such as pancreatic insufficiency
IV. Development of intestinal lymphoma
V. Development of diffuse intestinal ulceration
VI. Presence of nongranulomatous ulcerative jejunoileitis
VII. Presence of diffuse collagen deposits, i.e. "collagenous sprue"

III-9 BACTERIAL OVERGROWTH SYNDROMES

CONDITIONS ASSOCIATED WITH BACTERIAL OVERGROWTH

I. Billroth II subtotal gastrectomy with afferent loop stasis
II. Blind loops
III. Multiple small bowel diverticula
IV. Hypomotility states (diabetes, scleroderma, intestinal pseudo-obstruction)
V. Incomplete small bowel obstruction
VI. Gastric achlorhydria (pernicious anemia)
VII. Strictures (regional enteritis, radiation injury)
VIII. Fistulas (regional enteritis)

DIAGNOSIS OF "BACTERIAL OVERGROWTH" SYNDROME

*I. Steatorrhea—usually moderate (15-30 gm/day)
II. D-xylose—can be normal or abnormal
III. Small bowel biopsy—can be normal or abnormal
*IV. Vitamin B_{12} absorption with I.F.
*V. (+) Small bowel culture
  A. Usually > 10^7 organisms/ml
  B. Polymicrobial (E. coli, Bacteroides, enterococci, anaerobic lactobacilli)
VI. Abnormal breath tests (lactulose, ^{14}c-xylose, etc.)

* = Correction of #1, 4, and 5 with antibiotic therapy

III-I0 CLINICAL FEATURES OF ZINC DEFICIENCY*

Skin
  Acrodermatitis enteropathica
  Alopecia
  Poor wound healing
Neuropsychiatric
  Depression
  Irritability
  Lack of concentration
  Tremor

Gastrointestinal
  Anorexia
  Impaired taste
  Diarrhea
  Pancreatic insufficiency
Endocrinal
  Hypogonadism
  Dwarfism in children
  Insulin hypersensitivity
Eyes
  Night blindness

*From Advances in Internal Medicine. Vol. 26, 1980, p. 105.

III-11 DIFFERENTIAL DIAGNOSIS OF REGIONAL ENTERITIS

  I. Infectious enteritis (bacterial, fungal, protozoal)
    A. Must exclude amebiasis, campylobacter, yersinia
  II. Tuberculous enteritis
  III. Lymphoma
  IV. Carcinoid tumor
  V. Carcinoma
  VI. Intestinal lymphangiectasia
  VII. Ischemic small bowel disease with/without segmental infarcts
    A. Connective tissue disease with vasculitis (PN, SLE)
    B. Atherosclerotic/embolic disease
  VIII. Malabsorptive disorders with primary gut involvement
    A. Celiac sprue
    B. Amyloidosis
    C. Whipple's disease
  IX. Nongranulomatous ulcerative jejunoileitis
  X. Eosinophilic gastroenteritis

III-12 FEATURES DIFFERENTIATING IDIOPATHIC ULCERATIVE COLITIS FROM GRANULOMATOUS COLITIS*

Features	Ulcerative colitis	Granulomatous colitis
I. CLINICAL FEATURES		
Diarrhea	+ + + +	+ + +
Hematochezia	+ + + +	+ +
Abdominal tenderness	+ +	+ + +
Abdominal mass	0	+ + to + + +
Toxic megacolon	+	+
Perforation	+	+
Fistulas		
Perianal, perineal	0	+ +
Enteroenteric	0	+
II. ENDOSCOPIC FEATURES (SIGMOIDOSCOPY, COLONOSCOPY)		
Rectal involvement	+ + + +	+ +
Diffuse, continuous disease	+ + + +	+
Friability, purulence	+ + + to + + + +	+
Aphthous, linear ulcers	0	+ + + to + + + +
Cobblestoning	0	+ + to + + +
Pseudopolyps	+ +	+
III. RADIOLOGIC FEATURES		
Continuous disease	+ + + +	0 to +
Associated ileal disease	0	+ +
Strictures	0	+ to + +
Fistulas	0	+ to + +
Asymmetric wall involvement	0	+ + to + + +
Fissures	0	+ to + +
0		
IV. PATHOLOGIC FEATURES		
Granulomas	0	+ + + to + + + +
Transmural inflammation	0 to +	+ + + to + + + +
Crypt abscess	+ + +	+ to + +
Skip areas of involvement	0	+ + +
Linear, aphthous ulcers	0	+ + + to + + + +

*Key: 0 = never or rarely; + = ≤25%; + + = 25-50%; + + + = 50-75%; + + + + = >75%

Greenberger, N.J.: *Gastrointestinal Disorders: A Pathophysiological Approach*, 2nd Edition, Year Book Medical Publishers, Chicago, 1981, p. 217.

III-13 SYSTEMIC MANIFESTATIONS OF ULCERATIVE COLITIS (UC) AND REGIONAL ENTERITIS (RE)

	UC	RE
I. Skin		
A. Erythema nodosum	+	+
B. Pyoderma gangrenosum	+	+
C. Ulcerating erythematous plaques	+	+
II. Eyes		
A. Uveitis	+	+
III. Mouth		
A. Aphthous ulcers, chelitis	±	+
IV. Esophagus		
A. Ulceration	+	+
V. Stomach and Duodenum		
A. Pyloric outlet obstruction	−	+
VI. Small Bowel		
A. Malabsorption	−	+
B. Lactose intolerance	+	+
VII. Liver		
A. Steatosis	+	+
B. Cirrhosis	+	+
C. Chronic active liver disease	+	+
D. Granulomas	−	+
VIII. Gallbladder and Biliary Tree		
A. Cholelithiasis	−	+
B. Sclerosing cholangitis	+	rarely present
C. Bile duct carcinoma	+	−
IX. Renal Disease		
A. Obstructive hydronephrosis	−	+
B. Nephrolithiasis	+ (urate)	+ (oxalate)
X. Anemia		
A. Blood loss	+	+
B. Hemolysis	+	+
C. Folate depletion (Sulfasalazine)	+	+
D. Chronic illness	+	+
XI. Thrombocytosis	+	+
XII. Pulmonary		
A. Fibrosing alveolitis	+	−
B. Pulmonary vasculitis	+	−
XIII. Pancreatitis		
A. Ductal obstruction	−	+
B. Drugs (Azathioprine, sulfasalazine, steroids)	+	+
XIV. Vulva (Crohn's Disease)	−	+

CLASSIFICATION, DIAGNOSIS AND MANAGEMENT OF CHRONIC DIARRHEAL DISORDERS

Cause	Examples	Key Elements in Diagnosis	Treatment
1. Iatrogenic dietary factors	Excess tea, coffee, cola beverages, simple sugars	Careful history taking	Appropriate dietary modifications
2. Infectious enteritis	Amebiasis Giardiasis	Demonstrate leukocytes in stool Identify trophozoites or cysts in stool and duodenal aspirate (giardiasis)	Amebiasis—metronidazole diodoquin antibiotics Giardiasis—metronidazole
3. Inflammatory bowel disease	Ulcerative colitis Regional enteritis	History: diarrhea, abdominal pain, rectal bleeding Sigmoidoscopy, barium enema, UGI and small bowel series	Sulfadiazine Corticosteroids
4. Irritable bowel syndrome	See *Table IV*	See *Table IV*	Dietary modifications Antispasmodics See text
5. Lactose intolerance	Milk intolerance	Milk → abdominal pain, diarrhea, gas, bloating. Cessation of milk drinking → amelioration of symptoms Lactose load (1 gm/kg) → exacerbation of symptoms and blood glucose fails to rise > 20 mg/100 ml	Discontinue milk
6. Laxative abuse		Add few drops of NaOH to stool. Because most laxatives contain phenolphthalein, the stool will turn red.	Discontinue laxatives

7. Drug-induced	Antacids, antibiotics (clindamycin, lincomycin, amphicillin, penicillin), colchicine, PAS, lactulose, sorbitol	Careful history taking and review of medication.	D/C offending drug
8. Diverticular and prediverticular disease		History: intermittent symptoms P.E.: Palpable LF. colon Barium enema: diverticulosis and/or muscle hypertrophy	High fiber diet. Avoid: corn, nuts, peanuts, kernel-containing foods.
9. Malabsorptive disease	Sprue Pancreatic insufficiency	UGI plus small bowel x-rays; tests of intestinal absorptive function: D-xylose, stool fat, Schilling test, serum carotenes, calcium, albumin, cholesterol, iron, prothrombin time	Appropriate for the underlying disorder
10. Metabolic	Diabetes mellitus Hyperthyroidism Adrenal insufficiency	Abnormal blood glucose levels ↑ T4, ↑ RAI uptake ↓ plasma cortisol, ↓ response to synthetic ACTH	Appropriate to the underlying disorder
11. Mechanical	Fecal impaction	Rectal exam	Remove impaction
12. Neoplastic	Carcinoma of the pancreas Carcinoid syndrome Villous adenoma Medullary carcinoma of the thyroid Tumors producing V.I.P. (vasoactive intestinal peptide) Gastrinoma	Suspect the diagnosis	Surgical

Mnemonic to remember the classification: I, I, I, I, L, L, D, D, M, M, M, N

From: Greenberger, N.J., A Diagnostic Approach to the Patient with a Chronic Diarrheal Disorder. Journal of the Kansas Medical Society, June, 1978, pages 257-258.

III-15 DIAGNOSIS OF IRRITABLE BOWEL SYNDROME

I. Criteria useful in establishing the diagnosis
  A. Usual criteria
    1. Symptoms: Abdominal pain, diarrhea, alternating diarrhea and constipation, relief of abdominal pain with defecation, feeling of incomplete evacuation with defecation, absence of nocturnal symptoms.
    2. Absence of systemic symptoms: anorexia, weight loss, fever
    3. No hematochezia, melena, or occult blood in stool
    4. Normal sigmoidoscopy
    5. Normal barium enema
  B. Additional criteria if symptoms persist
    1. Normal stool weight (24 hr stool weight<300 gm)
    2. No steatorrhea or evidence of malabsorption
    3. Normal upper gastrointestinal tract and small bowel x-ray films
II. Differential diagnosis
  A. Lactose intolerance
  B. Other disaccharidase deficiencies, i.e. sucrose - isomaltose intolerance
  C. Subclinical carbohydrate malabsorption
  D. Diverticular and "prediverticular disease"
  E. Drug-induced diarrhea
  F. Idiopathic bile acid malabsorption
  G. Inadvertent dietary indiscretion (excess caffeine, tea, cola beverages, etc.)
  H. Irritable bowel disorder not associated with an underlying disorder

III-16 RISK FACTORS FOR DEVELOPING COLON CANCER

    I. Age > 40 years
   II. Family history of colon cancer
  III. Prior colon carcinoma
  IV. Familial polyposis
   V. Gardner's syndrome
  VI. Villous adenoma
 VII. Colonic polyps (especially if >2 cm)
VIII. Idiopathic ulcerative colitis
  IX. Granulomatous colitis (Crohn's disease)
   X. Prior breast or female genital tract cancer
  XI. Asbestosis
 XII. Diet rich in beef and lipid (controversial)
XIII. Cholecystectomy

Greenberger, N.J.: *Gastrointestinal Disorders: A Pathophysiological Approach*, 2nd Edition, Year Book Medical Publishers, Chicago, 1981, p. 227.

III-17 DIAGNOSIS OF CHRONIC ALCOHOLISM*

I. Evidence of alcohol withdrawal syndromes
   A. Tremulousness
   B. Alcoholic hallucinosis
   C. Withdrawal seizures or "rum fits"
   D. Delirium tremens
II. Evidence of tolerance to alcohol
   A. Ingestion of l fifth or more of whiskey per day
   B. No gross evidence of intoxication with blood alcohol level > 150 mg/100 ml
   C. Random blood alcohol level >300 mg/l00 ml
   D. Accelerated clearance of blood alcohol (>25 mg/100 ml per hour)
III. Psychosociologic factors
   A. Continued ingestion of alcohol despite strong contraindication to do so:
      1. Threatened loss of job
      2. Threatened loss of spouse and/or family
      3. Medical contraindication known to patient
   B. Admission of inability to discontinue use of alcohol
IV. Presence of alcohol-associated disorders
   A. Erosive gastritis with upper gastrointestinal bleeding
   B. Pancreatitis, acute and chronic, in the absence of cholelithiasis
   C. Alcoholic liver disease (fatty liver, alcoholic hepatitis, cirrhosis)
   D. Alcoholic diseases of the nervous system
      1. Peripheral neuropathy
      2. Cerebellar degeneration
      3. Wernicke-Korsakoff syndrome
      4. Beriberi
      5. Alcoholic myopathy
      6. Alcoholic cardiomyopathy

*Modified from Kaim, S.C., et al. *Ann. Intern. Med.* 77:249, 1972.

III-18 SPECTRUM OF ALCOHOLIC LIVER DISEASE

  I. Alcoholic fatty liver
- A. Clear cytoplasmic vacuoles
- B. Eccentrically placed cell nuclei

 II. Alcoholic hepatitis
- A. Polymorphonuclear infiltration
- B. Alcoholic hyaline
- C. Central hyaline necrosis and sclerosis of central vein
- D. Fat and/or fibrosis may be present

III. Alcoholic cirrhosis
- A. Distortion of lobular architecture
- B. Fibrous septa involve portal and central zones

IV. Secondary changes
- A. Cholestasis
- B. Bile duct proliferation
- C. Siderosis
- D. Fat

III-19 CLINICAL AND HISTOLOGICAL FEATURES OF ALCOHOLIC HEPATITIS

I. Clinical Features
   A. General considerations: Spectrum of clinical findings ranging from asymptomatic to florid decompensated liver disease with hepatosplenomegaly, jaundice, ascites, azotemia, and encephalopathy.
   B. Symptoms: Anorexia, weakness, abdominal pain, weight loss, fever
   C. Signs: Jaundice, peripheral stigmata of chronic liver disease, hepatomegaly, splenomegaly, ascites, edema, signs of hepatic encephalopathy
   D. Laboratory data: ↑ MCV, ↑ WBC, ↑ SGOT, ↑ SGOT:SGPT (AST:ALT)>3:1, ↑ bilirubin, ↓ albumin, prolonged prothrombin time
   E. Histologic features of alcoholic hepatitis
      1. Absolute criteria -
         a. Hepatocellular necrosis
         b. Polymorphonuclear infiltration of the liver
      2. Generally accepted criteria
         a. Mallory alcoholic hyaline
      3. Often present but not required for the diagnosis
         a. Fatty infiltration of the liver
         b. Fibrosis
         c. Cirrhosis
   F. Diagnosis of alcoholic hepatitis
      1. History of excessive alcohol intake
      2. Liver biopsy showing changes of alcoholic hepatitis
      3. Lab: ↑ MCV, ↑ SGOT, ↑ GGTP, ↑ SGOT:SGPT ratio
   G. Indicators of a bad prognosis
      1. Serum bilirubin >20 mg/dl
      2. BUN >25 mg/dl without obvious cause
      3. Hepatic encephalopathy
      4. Prothrombin time prolonged >6" compared to controls

———

III-20 HEPATITIS A

I. General Considerations
   A. Short incubation period (14-24 days)
   B. Fecal oral transmission (epidemics with contaminated water)
   C. Virus present in stools from incubation period to onset of clinical illness
   D. Triad of headache, fever, myalgias favors hepatitis A over hepatitis B
   E. Maximum period of infectivity 2 weeks after onset of clinical illness
   F. Frequently anicteric
   G. Does not result in chronic liver disease
   H. Infection confers immunity

II. Immunologic Considerations
   A. Hepatitis A antigen (Ha Ag) circulates transiently at low titers
   B. Ha Ag cleared rapidly from stool
   C. Ha Ag detection in serum and stool not feasible clinically
   D. Ha Ab rises rapidly, peaks after 2-3 months, persists
   E. Ha Ab in acute phase is IgM; later is IgG
   G. Ha Ab present in majority of adults (>50% at age >60)
   H. Conventional immune serum globulin *modifies* the disease

Greenberger, N.J.: *Gastrointestinal Disorders: A Pathophysiological Approach*, 2nd Edition, Year Book Medical Publishers, Chicago, 1981, p. 293.

LIVER

III-21 HEPATITIS B

EPIDEMIOLOGIC CONSIDERATIONS

Long incubation period (50 – 180 days)

Transmitted by parenteral and nonparenteral routes

Hb$_s$ Ag – spheres, tubules, Dane particles

Spheres and tubules represent viral surface coat material made in infected hepatocytes

Dane particle contains inner core antigen (Hb$_c$ Ag) and outer shell (Hb$_s$ Ag) and represents complete virion

Hb$_s$ Ag detected in blood, saliva, urine, semen, breast milk, bile

Sexual partners, homosexuals, and newborn infants have high rate of infection

IMMUNOLOGIC CONSIDERATIONS

Antigen	Significance
Hb$_s$ Ag	Hepatitis B infection
Hb$_c$ Ag	Hepatitis B infection
DNA polymerase	High infectivity; viral replication
Hb$_e$ Ag	Suggests high infectivity; associated with active disease

Antibody	Significance
Anti-Hb$_s$ (Hb$_s$ Ab)	Denotes prior hepatitis B infection and usually immunity
Anti-Hb$_c$ (Hb$_c$ Ab)	Recent or ongoing infection Hb$_s$ Ag carriers – high titers
Anti-Hb$_e$ (Hb$_e$ Ab)	Suggests limited/no disease activity/ and low-grade infectivity

DIAGNOSIS OF HEPATITIS B (HBV) INFECTION

Hb_s Ag positive in 75–85% of HBV infections
Reasons
   HBV present but below detectable concentrations
   HBV cleared, no Hb_s Ab (serologic window)
DX in Hb_s Ag negative patients established by demonstrating Hb_c Ab
(+) Hb_s Ag or other HBV markers in 30–40% chronic active liver disease patients

SPECTRUM OF RESPONSES IN HEPATITIS B INFECTIONS

Acute icteric hepatitis
   Serum bilirubin > 3.0 mg/dl
   Serum transaminases > 100 on > 2 occasions 4 days apart
Acute anicteric hepatitis
   Serum bilirubin < 3.0 mg/dl
   Serum transaminases > 100 on > 2 occasions 4 days apart
Seroconversion with Hb_s Ag positivity
   Hb_s Ag → Hb_s Ab
Seroconversion without Hb_s Ag positivity
   Hb_s Ab (−) → Hb_s Ab (+)

From Greenberger, N.J., Gastrointestinal Disorders. A Diagnostic Approach. 2nd Edition, 1981, page 294.

III-22 NON-A, NON-B HEPATITIS (NANBH)

I. Epidemiologic features
- A. At least 4 viruses
- B. Incubation period 6-14 weeks (mean, 7-8)
- C. NANBH antigen detectable 2-4 weeks (before enzyme increase
- D. Duration of antigenemia 2-12 weeks (mean, 8)
- E. Persistence of antigenemia correlated with SGPT elevations
- F. Clearance of antigen correlates with recovery and appearance of antibody
- G. NANBH antigen demonstrable in liver
- H. Virus characteristics by electron microscopy similar to hepatitis B virus
- I. Clinical settings
- J. Posttransfusion hepatitis (85-90% due to NANBH)
- K. Addicts (>50% episodes secondary to NANBH)
- L. Renal transplant patients
- M. Hemodialysis patients
- N. Multiply transfused hemophiliacs
  1. 50% have ↑ SGOT, SGPT
  2. 90% positive for Hb$_s$Ab
  3. Most bouts of hepatitis secondary to NANBH
- O. Bone marrow transplant patients
- P. Institutional outbreaks
- Q. Percutaneous transmission

II. Clinical Features
   A. NANBH is usually an anicteric, mildly symptomatic disease; probably undetected in most patients not prospectively followed
   B. Many cases associated with prolonged elevations of SGPT (40-50% >1 yr)
   C. Appreciable incidence of chronic active hepatitis and chronic persistent hepatitis
   D. 30% post NANBH vs. 10% post hepatitis B
III. Sequelae of Non-A, Non-B Hepatitis*
   A. 26/388 (6.7%) patients followed prospectively prior to open heart surgery developed NANBH
   B. 12/26 had elevated (often fluctuating) SGPT >1 year
   C. Liver biopsy done in 8/12; chronic active hepatitis found in 6, chronic persistent hepatitis in 2
   D. Risk of chronic active liver disease greatest in patients with anicteric hepatitis and SGPT >300
   E. Spontaneous improvement in 1-2 years in all 12 patients
IV. Conclusions
   A. Chronic active liver disease common sequela to acute NANBH
   B. Chronic active liver disease has better prognosis than from other causes

*Berman M., et al.: Ann. Intern. Med., 91:1, 1979. Greenberger, N.J.: *Gastrointestinal Disorders: A Pathophysiological Approach*, 2nd Edition, Year Book Medical Publishers, Chicago, 1981, p. 295.

III-23 ETIOLOGY AND DIAGNOSIS OF CHRONIC ACTIVE LIVER DISEASE

I. Causes of chronic active liver disease
   A. Autoimmune
   B. Viral hepatitis, type B
   C. Viral hepatitis, non-A, non-B (? 4 types)
   D. Drugs
      *1. Alpha methyl dopa
       2. Aspirin (esp. in patients with rheumatoid arthritis)
       3. Acetaminophen
       4. Allopurinol
       5. Halothane
      *6. Isoniazid
      *7. Nitrofurantoin
       8. Oxyphenisatin
       9. Propylthiouracil
      10. Sulfonamides
   E. Miscellaneous
       1. Wilson's disease
       2. Alpha-antitrypsin disease
II. Diagnosis of chronic active liver disease‡
   A. Persistence of symptoms and signs of liver disease for>6 months
   B. Persistence of abnormal liver tests for>6 months
       1. SGOT increased 10 times normal or
       2. SGOT increased 5 times normal and gammaglobulins increased 2 times normal
   C. Abnormal hepatic histology
       1. Chronic active hepatitis without cirrhosis
          a. periportal and piecemeal necrosis with portal zone expansion and rosette formation
          b. multilobular necrosis
          c. bridging (confluent) hepatic necrosis
          d. periportal plus piecemeal necrosis
       2. Chronic active hepatitis with cirrhosis

*Most important
‡Demonstration of ongoing activity for at least *6 months* emphasizes the unresolving nature of the process and is desirable for establishing the diagnosis. However, the onset of illness may be difficult to estimate. Thus, patients with disease of less than 6 months duration may develop hypoalbuminemia, hypergammaglobulinemia, and ascites and yet the disease is not fully chronic as judged by international criteria.

From Gastroenterology 70:1161, 1976.
From Mayo Clin. Proc. 56:311, 1981.

III-24 PRIMARY BILIARY CIRRHOSIS

I. Diagnosis
   A. Hepatomegaly
   B. ↑ Serum alkaline phosphatase
   C. (+) test for antimitochondrial antibody
   D. ↑ IgM levels
   E. ↑ Serum cholesterol
   F. Compatible histologic changes on liver biopsy
   G. Exclusion of extrahepatic obstruction

II. Natural history of primary biliary cirrhosis
   A. Hepatomegaly
   B. Pruritus
   C. Increased pigmentation
   D. Hyperbilirubinemia
   E. Xanthomata
   F. Splenomegaly
   G. Ascites
   H. G.I. bleeding

Appearance of clinical features as course of the disease progresses

III-25 COMMON PRECIPITATING CAUSES OF HEPATIC ENCEPHALOPATHY*

Cause	Possible Mechanisms Leading to Coma
I. Azotemia (spontaneous or diuretic-induced)	↑ BUN leads to ↑ endogenous NH_3 production; direct suppressive effect on brain from uremia
II. Sedatives, tranquilizers, anesthetics	Direct depressive effect on brain; impaired metabolism of sedative drugs with hepatic parenchymal cell failure
III. Gastrointestinal hemorrhage	Provides substrate for increased NH_3 production (100 ml blood = 15-20 gm protein)
	Shock and hypoxia
	Hypovolemia → impaired cerebral, hepatic, and renal function
	Azotemia can lead to further ↑ in blood NH_3 ↑ Load of NH_3 from transfused blood (Storage at 4 C: 1 day - 170 µg/100 ml; 4 days = 330; 21 days = 900.)
IV. Diuretics	Induce ↓ K^+ alkalosis ↓ K^+ leads to ↑ renal output NH_3 via renal veins Alkalosis leads to ↑ transfer of NH_3 across blood-brain barrier
	Vigorous diuresis can result in hypovolemia and impaired cardiac, cerebral, hepatic, and renal function, the latter resulting in azotemia; azotemia ↑ endogenous NH_3 production
V. Metabolic alkalosis	Favors transfer of nonionized NH_3 across blood-brain barrier

Cause	Possible Mechanisms Leading to Coma
VI. Increased dietary protein intake	Provides substrate for increased NH_3 production
VII. Infection	↑ Tissue catabolism leading to ↑ endogenous NH_3 load
	Dehydration and impaired renal function
	Hypoxia, hypotension, hyperthermia may potentiate NH_3 toxicity
VIII. Constipation	Intestinal production and absorption of NH_3 and other nitrogenous products
IX. Hepatic injury	Superimposed viral or toxic parenchymal cell injury may compromise liver function
X. Miscellaneous	N_4-containing drugs (NH_4Cl)
	Acquired form of renal tubular acidosis (distal type) with inappropriate kaliuresis
	Genetic disorders with specific deficiency of urea cycle enzymes
	Presence of hypoglycemia, hypercarbia, or severe hypoxemia in patients with marginal hepatocellular function

*Modified from: Schenker, S.: *Gastroenterology* 66:121, 1974, and Hoyumpa, A.M., Jr., et al.: *Gastroenterology* 76:184, 1979.

III-26 DIFFERENTIAL DIAGNOSIS OF ASCITES

I. Transudative effusions
   A. Cirrhosis of the liver*
   B. Congestive heart failure*
   C. Constrictive pericarditis*
   D. Obstruction to the hepatic veins (Budd-Chiari syndrome)*
      1. Associated with tumors (hepatoma, hypernephroma, cancer of pancreas)
      2. Associated with hematologic disorders (myeloproliferative disease, polycythemia vera, myeloid metaplasia)
      3. Due to infections (pylephlebitis)
   E. Obstruction to the inferior vena cava
   F. Nephrotic syndrome
   G. Viral hepatitis with submassive or massive hepatic necrosis
   H. Meig's syndrome

II. Exudative effusions
   A. Neoplastic diseases involving the peritoneum*
      1. Peritoneal carcinomatosis
      2. Lymphomatous disorders
   B. Tuberculous peritonitis*
   C. Pancreatitis* (also leaking pseudocyst and disrupted main pancreatic duct)
   D. Talc or starch powder peritonitis following surgery
   E. Transected lymphatics following portal-caval shunt surgery
   F. Myxedema
   G. Sarcoidosis
   H. Lymphatic obstruction
      1. Intestinal lymphangiectasia
      2. Lymphomas
   I. Pseudomyxoma peritonei
   J. Struma ovarii
   K. Amyloidosis
   L. Prior abdominal trauma with ruptured lymphatics
   M. Nephrogenic ascites¶

III. Disorders simulating ascites
   A. Pancreatic pseudocyst
   B. Hydronephrosis
   C. Ovarian cyst
   D. Mesenteric cyst
   E. Obesity

* Most common disorders.
¶ Occurs in patients with renal failure on maintenance hemodialysis.

Greenberger, N.J.: *Gastrointestinal Disorders: A Pathophysiological Approach*, 2nd Edition, Year Book Medical Publishers, Chicago, 1981, p. 336.

III-27 CONDITIONS CAUSING OR CONTRIBUTING TO POSTOPERATIVE JAUNDICE*

I. Increased load of bilirubin pigment
   A. Hemolytic anemia
   B. Resorption of hematomas or hemoperitoneum
   C. Pulmonary infarction
   D. Transfusions: If blood stored >1 week, approximately 10% of red blood cells hemolyzed → extra load of ~ 7.5 gm hemoglobin. $7.5 \times 35 = ~ 250$ mg extra bilirubin/unit blood

II. Impaired hepatocellular function
   A. Hepatitis-like picture
     1. Posttransfusion hepatitis
       a. Non-A, non-B hepatitis (85-90%)
       b. Hepatitis B (10-15%)
       c. Cytomegalovirus, EB virus, adenovirus, ECHO, coxsackie (<5%)
     2. Hypotension
     3. Halothane anesthesia
     4. Drugs
   B. Intrahepatic cholestasis
     1. Hypotension
     2. Hypoxemia
     3. Sepsis
     4. Drugs
     5. Total parenteral nutrition
   C. Congestive heart failure

III. Extrahepatic biliary tract obstruction
   A. Bile duct injury
   B. Choledocholithiasis

Modified from LaMont, J.F., and Isselbacher, K.J.: N. Engl. J. Med. 288:305, 1973.

———

III-28 DIFFERENTIAL DIAGNOSIS OF INTRAHEPATIC CHOLESTASIS*

I. Hepatocellular
   A. Viral hepatitis
   B. Alcoholic hepatitis
   C. Chronic active hepatitis
II. Hepatocanalicular
   A. Drugs (17-alkylated steroids, phenothiazines)
   B. Sepsis
   C. Toxic shock syndrome
   D. Postoperative
   E. Total parenteral nutrition
   F. Neoplasms (Hodgkin's disease, lymphoma, prostatic carcinoma)
   G. Sickle cell anemia
   H. Amyloidosis
III. Ductular
   A. Sarcoidosis
   B. Primary biliary cirrhosis
IV. Ducts
   A. Intrahepatic biliary atresia
   B. Intrahepatic sclerosing cholangitis
   C. Caroli's disease
   D. Cholangiocarcinoma
V. Recurrent cholestasis
   A. Benign recurrent intrahepatic cholestasis
   B. Recurrent jaundice of pregnancy
   C. Dubin Johnson syndrome

* Classification based on apparent site of hepatic injury.

III-29 DIFFERENTIAL DIAGNOSIS OF IRON STORAGE DISEASE AND CLINICAL FEATURES OF IDIOPATHIC HEMOCHROMATOSIS

	Iron overload in family members	Anemia	Cirrhosis	Transferrin saturation	Serum ferritin	Desferrioxamine iron excretion
I. Refractory anemias	0	+	0	Normal-↑	Variable	Variable
II. Laennec's cirrhosis	0	±	+	Normal−	Normal-↑	2-4 mg/24 hr
III. Excess oral iron intake	0	±	0	↑	Normal-↑	Variable
IV. Transfusion hemosiderosis	0	+	0	↑	↑	Variable
V. Idiopathic hematochromsatosis*	+	0	±	>80%	>1,000 ng/ml	>8 mg/24 hr

    A. Skin pigmentation
    B. Diabetes mellitus
    C. Hepatomegaly, splenomegaly, cirrhosis
    D. Hypogonadism
    E. Cardiomyopathy and congestive heart failure
    F. Adrenal insufficiency
    G. Arthropathy

+ = present; 0 = absent; ± = may or may not be present.

* Liver biopsy shows parenchymal distribution of iron deposits.

Greenberger, N.J.: *Gastrointestinal Disorders: A Pathophysiological Approach*, 2nd Edition, Year Book Medical Publishers, Chicago, 1981, p. 357.

III-30 COMPARISON OF THE CLINICAL, RADIOLOGIC, AND PATHOLOGIC CHARACTERISTICS OF FOCAL NODULAR HYPERPLASIA AND LIVER CELL ADENOMA*

	Focal Nodular Hyperplasia	Liver Cell Adenoma
I. Clinical		
Incidence	Uncommon	Rare
Age	All ages	Third, fourth decades
Sex	85% F	Nearly all F
Oral contraceptive use	Occasionally	Nearly always
Clinical presentation	Usually asymptomatic; 35% have abdominal mass, abdominal discomfort	Often abdominal emergency, 45% abdominal mass, acute abdominal pain
Hemoperitoneum	Less than 1%	25%
Liver function tests	Nearly always normal	Nearly always normal
Malignant potential	Resection if operative risk negligible	Resection
II. Angiography		
Vascularity	Hypervascular with dense capillary blush	Hypovascular
Hematoma formation	Rare	Common
Necrosis	Rare	Common
Septation	Present in 50%	Absent
III. Liver scan		
Uptake	Normal or slightly decreased	None
IV. Pathology		
Capsule	No capsule	Partial to ample encapsulation
Location	Usually subcapsular, 20% pedunculated	Usually subcapsular, 7% pedunculated
Lesions	Often multiple	Usually solitary
Stellate scar	Present	Absent
Parenchyma	Nodular	Homogeneous
Hemorrhage, necrosis	Rare	Common
Bile stasis	Absent	Present
Hepatocytes	Cytologically normal	Glycogen rich, vacuolated
Bile ductules	Present	Absent
Kupffer cells	Present	Reduced or absent
Vascularity	Large thick-walled vessels	Thin-walled sinusoids
Ultrastructure	Normal	Simplified

*Modified from: Knowles, D.M., II, et al: Medicine 57:223, 1978.

III-31 CLINICAL FEATURES OF HEPATOMA

I. Generally 80-90% of primary hepatic neoplasms are hepatic cell carcinomas (i.e., hepatoma); 10% are bile duct carcinomas (cholangiocarcinoma); approximately 70% of patients have underlying cirrhosis, most frequently postnecrotic or "mixed" type

II. Symptoms
   A. Common: weight loss, abdominal pain, anorexia, nausea, and emesis, which occur in 40-70% of patients
   B. Uncommon: fever, cough, hemoptysis

III. Physical findings
   A. Common: hepatomegaly, ascites, jaundice, hepatic bruit, liver tenderness to palpation, edema
   B. Uncommon: splenomegaly, hepatic coma (except terminally), fever

IV. Atypical presentations and manifestations
   A. Acute cholecystitis syndrome
   B. Acute abdominal catastrophe (hemoperitoneum)
   C. Pulmonary embolism with or without infarction and malignant pleural effusion
   D. Budd-Chiari syndrome
   E. Erythrocytosis (~ 10% of patients)
   F. Hypercalcemia
   G. Hypoglycemia
   H. Hypercholesterolemia
   I. Fever of unknown origin

V. Diagnosis
   A. Clinical findings
      1. Unexplained deterioration in a cirrhotic*
      2. Hepatomegaly with a disproportionately serum alkaline phosphatase with no or little elevation in serum bilirubin*
      3. Hepatic bruit
      4. Elevated right diaphragm

VI. Laboratory findings
   A. Abnormal liver scan/sonogram/CT scan
   B. Abnormal hepatic angiogram*
   C. Abnormal fibrinogen
   D. Positive liver biopsy (approximately 70% of cases)*
   E. Distant metastases

VII. Serologic tumor markers
   A. Alphafetoprotein (70-85% of cases)
   B. Hepatitis B markers in serum and liver (42-88% of cases)
   C. Vitamin B_{12} binding protein (7% of cases)
   D. Alpha-$_1$-antitrypsin (5% of cases)
   E. Immunoreactive calcitonin (?90% of cases)

(continued)

III-31 CLINICAL FEATURES OF HEPATOMA (CONTINUED)

VIII. Course
- A. Average course is 4-8 months after onset of symptoms
- B. Generally poor responses to chemotherapy
- C. Gastrointestinal bleeding is common (35%-50% of cases)
- D. Hepatic coma develops in 20-30% of cases

*Most important

Greenberger, N.J.: *Gastrointestinal Disorders: A Pathophysiological Approach*, 2nd Edition, Year Book Medical Publishers, Chicago, 1981, p. 361.

III-32 DIAGNOSIS OF WILSON'S DISEASE

I. Abnormalities uniformly present
- *A. Kayser-Fleischer rings
- *B. Serum ceruloplasmin (> 20 mg/100 ml)
- *C. Urine copper excretion (120 μg/day)
- D. Liver copper content (> 250 μg/gm dry wt. of liver)
- E. Abnormal metabolism of ^{64}Cu

II. Abnormalities frequently present
- A. Serum uric acid and uricosuria
- B. Aminoaciduria
- C. Renal glycosuria
- D. Chronic active liver disease, cirrhosis
- E. Splenomegaly
- F. Thrombocytopenia
- G. Hemolytic anemia

III. Central nervous system abnormalities

Greenberger, N.J.: *Gastrointestinal Disorders: A Pathophysiological Approach*, 2nd Edition, Year Book Medical Publishers, Chicago, 1981, p. 359.
* = These 3 items are used to screen for Wilson's disease.

III-33 COMPLICATIONS OF CORTICOSTEROID THERAPY

  I. Stigmata of hypercorticism
- A. Acne
- B. Hirsutism
- C. Moon facies
- D. Cervico-thoracic obesity
- E. Striae
- F. Easy bruisability
- G. Impaired wound healing

  II. Problems secondary to abnormalities in salt and water metabolism
- A. Sodium retention
- B. Weight gain (also increased appetite and polyphagia)
- C. Edema
- D. Increased blood pressure
- E. Hypokalemia (muscle weakness)

  III. Endocrine-metabolic problems
- A. Unmask latent diabetes
- B. Aggravate manifest diabetes
- C. Potential for adrenal crises with abrupt discontinuation of Rx or stress

  IV. Musculo-skeletal
- A. Steroid myopathy with muscle weakness
- B. Osteopenia
- C. Compression fractures
- D. Aseptic necrosis femoral head

  V. Gastrointestinal
- A. Vague abdominal pain
- B. Dyspepsia
- C. ? ↑ likelihood of peptic ulcer
- D. ? ↑ likelihood of G.I. bleeding
- E. Pancreatitis
- F. Mask an acute abdomen

(continued)

III-33 COMPLICATIONS OF CORTICOSTEROID THERAPY (CONTINUED)

VI. Nervous system
   A. Depression
   B. Euphoria
   C. Insomnia
   D. Irritability
   E. Psychosis

VII. Hematologic
   A. Leukocytosis
   B. Neutrophilia
   C. Lymphocytopenia

VIII. Immunologic—Infectious
   A. False negative skin tests
   B. Increased susceptibility to infections
   C. Opportunistic infections
   D. Reactivation of tuberculosis
   E. Impaired cell mediated immunity

IX. Miscellaneous
   A. Premature cataracts

III-34 LYMPHORETICULAR MALIGNANCY PRESENTING AS FULMINANT HEPATIC DISEASE*

I. Clinical presentation
   A. Fever, malaise, nausea, vomiting, abdominal pain
   B. Jaundice with progressive hyperbilirubinemia
   C. Hepatic failure, renal failure, coagulation abnormalities
   D. Absence of lymphadenopathy and splenomegaly
   E. Clinical course with death in 2-4 weeks after hospitalization
   F. Pathology: malignant histocytosis or primitive lymphoreticular malignancy

*From Gastroenterology, 82:339, 1982.

III-35 CAUSES OF ACUTE PANCREATITIS*

   I. Alcohol ingestion (acute and chronic alcoholism)
  II. Biliary tract disease (gallstones)
 III. Postoperative (abdominal, nonabdominal)
  IV. Post-endoscopic retrograde cholangiopancreatography (ERCP)
   V. Trauma (especially blunt abdominal trauma)
  VI. Metabolic
      A. Hypertriglyceridemia
      B. Hyperparathyroidism
      C. Renal failure
      D. Acute fatty liver of pregnancy
 VII. Hereditary pancreatitis
VIII. Infections
      A. Mumps
      B. Viral hepatitis
      C. Mycoplasma
      D. Other viral infections (coxsackie and ECHO virus)
  IX. Connective tissue disorders with vasculitis
      A. Systemic lupus erythematosus
      B. Necrotizing angiitis
      C. Thrombotic thrombocytopenic purpura
      D. Henoch Schönlein purpura
   X. Drug associated
      A. Definite association
         1. Azathioprine
         2. Sulfonamides
         3. Thiazide diuretics
         4. Furosemide
         5. Estrogens (oral contraceptives)
         6. Tetracycline
         7. Valproic acid

(Continued)

III-35   CAUSES OF ACUTE PANCREATITIS (CONTINUED)

B. Probable association
1. Chlorthalidone
2. Ethacrynic acid
3. Procainamide
4. L-asparaginase
5. Iatrogenic hypercalcemia
6. Methyl dopa
C. Equivocal association
1. Corticosteroids
XI. Obstruction of the ampulla of vater
A. Regional enteritis
B. Duodenal diverticulum
XII. Penetrating duodenal ulcer
XIII. Pancreas divisum
XIV. Recurrent bouts of acute pancreatitis without obvious cause
A. Consider
1. Occult disease of the gallbladder, biliary tree, pancreas, pancreatic ducts
2. Drugs
3. Hypertriglyceridemia
4. Pancreas divisum
5. Hereditary pancreatitis

* Adapted from: Greenberger, N.J., Toskes, P., and Isselbacher, K.J.: Diseases of the Pancreas, in *Harrison's Principles of Internal Medicine*, 10th Edition, McGraw-Hill Book Company, New York City, 1983 (in press).

III-36 FACTORS ADVERSELY INFLUENCING SURVIVAL IN ACUTE PANCREATITIS*

I. Risk factors identifiable upon admission to hospital
   A. Increasing age
   B. Hypotension
   C. Tachycardia
   D. Abnormal physical examination of the lungs
   E. Abdominal mass
   F. Fever
   G. Leukocytosis
   H. Hyperglycemia
   I. First attack of pancreatitis

II. Risk factors identifiable during initial 48 hr of hospitalization
   A. Fall in hematocrit > 10% with hydration and/or hematocrit < 30%
   B. Necessity for massive fluid and colloid replacement
   C. Hypocalcemia
   D. Hypoxemia with or without adult respiratory distress syndrome
   E. Hypoalbuminemia
   F. Azotemia

III. Major risk factors[+]
   1. Hypotension
   2. Need for massive fluid and colloid replacement
   3. Respiratory failure
   4. Hypocalcemia

* Increased mortality can be expected if 3 or more risk factors in Groups I and II are present.

+ If 3 or more major risk factors from group III are present, mortality rates can be expected to be as high as 65%.

Adapted from: Jacobs, M.L., et al., Ann. Surg. *185*:43-51, 1977, and Ranson, J.H.C., et al., J. Surg. Res., *22*:79-91, 1977.

III-37 COMPLICATIONS OF ACUTE PANCREATITIS*

I. Local
  A. Pancreatic phlegmon
  B. Pancreatic pseudocyst
     1. Pain
     2. Rupture with/without hemorrhage
     3. Hemorrhage
     4. Infection
  C. Pancreatic ascites
     1. Disruption of main pancreatic duct
     2. Leaking pseudocyst
  D. Pancreatic abscess
  E. Involvement of contiguous organs by necrotizing pancreatitis
     1. Massive intraperitoneal hemorrhage
     2. Thrombosis of blood vessels
     3. Bowel infarction
  F. Obstructive jaundice

II. Systemic
  A. Pulmonary
     1. Atelectasis
     2. Pneumonitis
     3. Pleural effusion
     4. Mediastinal abscess
     5. Adult respiratory distress syndrome
  B. Cardiovascular
     1. Hypotension
        a. hypovolemia
        b. hypoalbuminemia
     2. Sudden death
     3. Nonspecific ST-T changes in electrocardiogram simulating myocardial infarction
     4. Pericardial effusion
  C. Hematologic
     1. Disseminated intravascular coagulation (DIC)
  D. Gastrointestinal hemorrhage
     1. Peptic ulcer disease
     2. Erosive gastritis
     3. Hemorrhagic pancreatic necrosis with erosion into major blood vessels
     4. Portal vein thrombosis; variceal hemorrhage
  E. Renal
     1. Oliguria (usually due to hypovolemia)
     2. Azotemia (usually due to hypovolemia)
     3. Renal artery and/or renal vein thrombosis
  F. Metabolic
     1. Hyperglycemia
     2. Hypertriglyceridemia
     3. Hypocalcemia

III-37 COMPLICATIONS OF ACUTE PANCREATITIS (CONTINUED)

    G. Central nervous system
        1. Psychosis
        2. Fat emboli
        3. Encephalopathy
    H. Fat necrosis
        1. Subcutaneous tissues/erythematosus nodules
        2. Bone
        3. Other organs (mediastinum, pleura, nervous system)
    I. Miscellaneous
        1. Sudden blindness (Purtscher's retinopathy)

* Adapted from: Greenberger, N.J., Toskes, P., and Isselbacher, K.J.: Diseases of the Pancreas. in *Harrison's Principles of Internal Medicine*, 10th Edition, McGraw-Hill Book Company, New York, City, 1983 (in press).

III-38 COMPLICATIONS OF CHRONIC PANCREATITIS

    I. Exocrine pancreatic insufficiency, steatorrhea, creatorrhea
    II. Vitamin B_{12} malabsorption
    III. Diabetes mellitus (difficult to exclude genetic diabetes)
    IV. Recurrent bouts of acute pancreatitis
    V. Pleural effusion (usually left-sided)
    VI. Pericardial effusion (rare)
    VII. Pancreatic ascites
        A. Disruption of pancreatic duct
        B. Leaking pseudocyst
    VIII. Altered mental status (psychosis, etc.)
    IX. Ischemic necrosis of bone and intramedullary calcification
    X. Common bile duct stenosis, obstructive jaundice, biliary cirrhosis
    XI. Addiction to narcotics and analgesics
    XII. ? Increased incidence of pancreatic carcinoma

III-39 DIAGNOSIS OF EXOCRINE PANCREATIC INSUFFICIENCY (E.P.I.)

I. Identify etiology of E.P.I.
II. Steatorrhea* with/without creatorrhea; ↑ stool N_2
III. Pancreatic calcification*
IV. Diabetes mellitus*
V. Test of pancreatic exocrine function[+]
   A. Secretin with/without CCK-PZ → ↓ volume, [HCO_3], ↓ enzyme output
   B. Tripeptide test (Bentiromide) → ↓ urine excretion of Para-aminobenzoic acid (PABA)
VI. ↓ Absorption of vitamin B_{12}
VII. Normal tests of mucosal function (D-xylose, small bowel mucosal biopsy)
VIII. Response to pancreatic enzyme therapy
   A. Weight gain
   B. ↓ steatorrhea, creatorrhea

*Classical diagnostic—triad

+Frequently necessary as only 1/4 patients with exocrine pancreatic insufficiency have the classical diagnostic triad

IV—Hematology-Oncology

IV-1 DIFFERENTIAL DIAGNOSIS OF NORMOCHROMIC-NORMOCYTIC ANEMIA

I. Primary bone marrow failure
   A. Aplastic anemia
   B. Myelophthisic anemia
      1. Leukemia and lymphoma
      2. Other neoplasms
      3. Myelofibrosis
      4. Granulomas
II. Secondary anemias
   A. Anemia of chronic inflammation
      1. Connective tissue disease
      2. Chronic infection
   B. Anemia of uremia
   C. Anemias associated with endocrinopathies
      1. Hypothyroidism
      2. Addison's disease
      3. Hypogonadism
      4. Panhypopituitarism
   D. Anemia associated with chronic liver disease

Modified from: Bunn, H.F.: in *Harrison's Principles of Internal Medicine*, Isselbacher, K.J., Adams, R.D., Braunwald, E., Petersdorf, R.G., and Wilson, J.D. (eds.), 9th Edition, McGraw-Hill Book Company, New York City, 1980, p. 269.

IV-2 DIFFERENTIAL DIAGNOSIS OF MICROCYTIC-HYPOCHROMIC ANEMIA

I. Iron deficiency anemia
   A. Blood loss
   B. Insufficient iron in the diet
   C. Impaired absorption
   D. Increased requirements
II. Sideroblastic anemia
   A. Hereditary or congenital
      1. X-linked
      2. Autosomal recessive
   B. Acquired sideroblastic anemia
      1. Idiopathic refractory sideroblastic anemia
      2. Secondary to underlying disease A
         a. neoplasms
         b. inflammatory
         c. hematologic
         d. metabolic
      3. Associated with drugs or toxins
         a. ethanol
         b. lead
         c. antituberculosis agents
         d. chloramphenicol
         e. antineoplastic agents
III. Thalassemia

Modified from: Lee, G.R., Wintrobe, M.M., Bunn, H.F.: in *Harrison's Principles of Internal Medicine*, Isselbacher, K.J., Adams, R.D., Braunwald, E., Petersdorf, R.G., and Wilson, J.D. (eds.), 9th Edition, McGraw-Hill Book Company, New York City, 1980, p. 1515, 1517.

IV-3 DIFFERENTIAL DIAGNOSIS OF MACROCYTIC ANEMIAS

I. Vitamin B_{12} deficiency
   A. Inadequate intake
   B. Malabsorption
      1. Low intrinsic factor
         a. pernicious anemia
         b. postgastrectomy
         c. congenital absence of intrinsic factor
      2. Disorders of terminal ileum
         a. surgical resection
         b. sprue
         c. inflammatory bowel disease
         d. neoplasms
      3. Competition for vitamin B_{12}
         a. fish tapeworm
         b. bacteria: blind loop syndrome
      4. Drugs
         a. p-aminosalicylic acid
         b. colchicine
         c. neomycin
   C. Transcobalamin II deficiency

II. Folate deficiency
   A. Inadequate intake
   B. Malabsorption
   C. Increased requirements
      1. Pregnancy
      2. Infancy
      3. Malignancy
      4. Chronic hemolytic anemia
   D. Impaired metabolism
      1. Methotrexate and other drugs that inhibit dihydrofolate reductase
      2. Alcohol
      3. Enzyme deficiencies

III. Miscellaneous
   A. Chemotherapeutic agents which interfere with DNA metabolism
      1. 6-mercaptopurine
      2. Azathioprine
      3. 5-Fluorouracil
      4. Cytosine arabinoside
      5. Procarbazine
      6. Hydroxyurea
   B. Hereditary orotic aciduria and other rare metabolic disorders
   C. Megaloblastic anemias of unknown etiology
      1. Refractory megaloblastic anemia
      2. DiGuglielmo's syndrome

Modified from: Babior, B.M., Bunn, H.F.: in *Harrison's Principles of Internal Medicine*, Isselbacher, K.J., Adams, R.D., Braunwald, E., Petersdorf, R.G., and Wilson, J.D. (eds.), 9th Edition, McGraw-Hill Book Company, New York City, 1980, p. 1519.

IV-4 DIFFERENTIAL DIAGNOSIS OF HEMOLYTIC ANEMIAS

I. Inherited disorders
- A. Defects in the erythrocyte membrane
    1. Hereditary spherocytosis
    2. Hereditary eliptocytosis
- B. Deficiency of erythrocyte glycolytic enzymes
    1. Pyruvate kinase
    2. Hexokinase
- C. Abnormalities of erythrocyte nucleotide metabolism
    1. Pyrimidine 5'nucleotidase deficiency
    2. Adenosine deaminase excess
- D. Deficiencies of enzymes involved in the pentose phosphate pathway and in glutathione metabolism
    1. G-6PD
    2. Glutamyl-cysteine synthetase
- E. Defects in globin structure and synthesis
    1. Sickle cell anemia
    2. Thalassemia

II. Acquired disorders
- A. Immunohemolytic anemias
    1. Secondary to transfusion of incompatible blood
    2. Hemolytic disease of the newborn
    3. Due to warm reactive antibodies
        a. idiopathic
        b. "secondary"
            (1) virus and mycoplasma infection
            (2) lymphosarcoma and CLL
            (3) other malignancies
            (4) immune-deficiency states
            (5) systemic lupus erythematosus and other "autoimmune" disorders
        c. drug induced
    4. Due to cold reactive antibodies
        a. cold hemagglutinin disease
        b. paroxysmal cold hemoglobinuria
- B. Traumatic and microangiopathic hemolytic anemias
    1. Prosthetic values and other cardiac abnormalities
    2. Hemolytic-uremic syndrome
    3. Thrombotic thrombocytopenic purpura
    4. Disseminated intravascular coagulation
    5. Graft rejection
    6. Immune complex disease

    C. Infectious agents
- 1. Protozoan
  - a. malaria
  - b. toxoplasmosis
  - c. leishmaniasis
  - d. trypanosomiasis
- 2. Bacterial
  - a. bartonellosis
  - b. clostridial infections
  - c. typhoid fever

    D. Chemicals, drugs and venoms
- 1. Oxidant drugs and chemicals
  - a. napthalene
  - b. nitrofurantoin
  - c. sulfonamides
- 2. Non-oxidant chemicals
  - a. arsine
  - b. copper
  - c. water
- 3. Associated with hemodialysis and uremia
- 4. Venoms

    E. Physical agents
- 1. Thermal injury
- 2. (?) ionizing radiation

    F. Hypophosphatemia

    G. "Spur cell" anemia in liver disease

    H. Paroxysmal nocturnal hemoglobinuria

    I. Vitamin E deficiency in newborns

Modified from: Wintrobe, M.M. et al.: in *Clinical Hematology*, Eighth Edition, Lea & Febiger, Philadelphia, 1981, p. 737.

IV-5 DIFFERENTIAL DIAGNOSIS OF APLASTIC ANEMIA

    I. Idiopathic
    II. Constitutional (Fanconi's anemia)
    III. Chemical and physical agents
        A. Dose-related
            1. Chloramphenicol
            2. Benzene
            3. Ionizing irradiation
            4. Alkylating agents
            5. Antimetabolites (folic acid antagonists, purine and pyrimidine analogues)
            6. Mitotic inhibitors
            7. Anthracyclines
            8. Inorganic arsenicals
        B. Idiosyncratic
            1. Chloramphenicol
            2. Phenylbutazone
            3. Sulfa drugs
            4. Methylphenylethylhydantoin
            5. Gold compounds
            6. Organic arsenicals
            7. Insecticides
    IV. Hepatitis
    V. Immunologically mediated aplasia
    VI. Pregnancy
    VII. Paroxysmal nocturnal hemoglobinuria
    VIII. Miscellaneous: Systemic lupus erythematosus, pancreatitis, miliary tuberculosis, Simmonds' disease, viral infections

Adapted from: Rappeport, J.M, Bunn, H.F.: in *Harrison's Principles of Internal Medicine*, Isselbacher, K.J., Adams, R.D., Braunwald, E., Petersdorf, R.G., and Wilson, J.D. (eds.), 9th Edition, McGraw-Hill Book Company, New York City, 1980, p. 1526.

IV-6 DIFFERENTIAL DIAGNOSIS OF PANCYTOPENIA

    I. Aplastic anemia
    II. Pancytopenia with normal or increased bone marrow cellularity
        A. Idiopathic refractory anemia
        B. Hypersplenism
        C. Vitamin B_{12} or folate deficiency
        D. Paroxysmal nocturnal hemoglobinuria (variable cellularity)
        E. Connective tissue disorders (SLE)
        F. Sarcoidosis

III. Bone marrow replacement
   A. Hematologic malignancies
   B. Nonhematologic metastatic tumor
   C. Storage-cell disorders
   D. Osteopetrosis
   E. Myelofibrosis

Adapted from: Rappeport, J.M., Bunn, H.F.: in *Harrison's Principles of Internal Medicine*, Isselbacher, K.J., Adams, R.D., Braunwald, E., Petersdorf, R.G., and Wilson, J.D. (eds.), 9th Edition, McGraw-Hill Book Company, New York City, 1980, p. 1525.

IV-7 DIFFERENTIAL DIAGNOSIS OF NEUTROPENIA

I. Hematologic diseases
   A. Chronic idiopathic neutropenia
   B. Cyclic neutropenia
   C. Leukemia
   D. Chediak-Higashi syndrome
   E. Aplastic anemia
II. Drug-induced conditions
   A. Agranulocytosis
   B. Myelotoxic drugs
III. Nutritional deficiencies
   A. Vitamin B_{12}
   B. Folate
   C. Copper
IV. Secondary to other diseases
   A. Infections
      1. Typhoid
      2. Mononucleosis
      3. Malaria
      4. Overwhelming sepsis
   B. Diseases with splenomegaly
      1. Felty's syndrome
      2. Congestive splenomegaly
      3. Gaucher's disease
      4. Sarcoidosis
   C. Malignancies with marrow invasion

Modified from: Dale, D.C.: in *Harrison's Principles of Internal Medicine*, Isselbacher, K.J., Adams, R.D., Braunwald, E., Petersdorf, R.G., and Wilson, J.D. (eds.), 9th Edition, McGraw-Hill Book Company, New York City, 1980, p. 286.

IV-8 DIFFERENTIAL DIAGNOSIS OF NEUTROPHILIA

   I. Physiologic
      A. Exercise
      B. Epinephrine
      C. Pain, emotion, or stress
  II. Infections
      A. Bacterial
      B. Parasitic
      C. Fungal
      D. Viral (less common)
 III. Inflammation
      A. Burns
      B. Tissue necrosis
         1. Myocardial infarction
         2. Pulmonary infarction
      C. Connective tissue disease
  IV. Metabolic disorders
      A. Diabetic ketoacidosis
      B. Acute renal failure
      C. Eclampsia
      D. Poisoning
   V. Myeloproliferative diseases
  VI. Miscellaneous
      A. Metastatic carcinoma
      B. Acute hemorrhage or hemolysis
      C. Glucocorticosteroids
      D. Lithium therapy
      E. Idiopathic

Modified from: Dale, D.C.: in *Harrison's Principles of Internal Medicine*, Isselbacher, K.J., Adams, R.D., Braunwald, E., Petersdorf, R.G., and Wilson, J.D. (eds.), 9th Edition, McGraw-Hill Book Company, New York City, 1980, p. 286.

IV-9 DIFFERENTIAL DIAGNOSIS OF EOSINOPHILIA

   I. Allergic disorders
      A. Hay fever
      B. Asthma
      C. Urticaria
      D. Some instances of drug sensitivity

II. Dermatologic disorders including:
   A. Pemphigus
   B. Dermatitis herpetiformis
III. Parasitic infections
   A. Trichinosis
   B. Echinococcus
IV. Pulmonary infiltrate with eosinophilia
V. Malignancy
   A. Hodgkin's disease
   B. Chronic myelogenous leukemia
   C. Mycosis fungoides
   D. Pernicious anemia
   E. Polycythemia vera
   F. Malignant disease of any type, usually associated with metastases or necrosis
VI. Connective tissue disease
   A. Rheumatoid arthritis
   B. Dermatomyositis
   C. Periarteritis nodosa
VII. Hypereosinophilic syndromes
VIII. Sarcoidosis
IX. Miscellaneous
   A. Adrenal insufficiency
X. Idiopathic

Modified from: Dale, D.C.: in *Harrison's Principles of Internal Medicine*, Isselbacher, K.J., Adams, R.D., Braunwald, E., Petersdorf, R.G., and Wilson, J.D. (eds.), 9th Edition, McGraw-Hill Book Company, New York City, 1980, p. 290.

IV-10 DIFFERENTIAL DIAGNOSIS OF BASOPHILIA

I. Hematologic disorders
   A. Hodgkin's disease
   B. Polycythemia vera
   C. Chronic myelogenous leukemia
   D. Myelofibrosis
II. Chronic inflammatory conditions
   A. Ulcerative colitis
   B. Chronic sinusitis
   C. Occasionally with nephrosis
III. Myxedema

Modified from: Wintrobe, M.M. et al: in *Clinical Hematology*, Eighth Edition, Lea & Febiger, Philadelphia, 1981, p. 1300-1301.

IV-11 DIFFERENTIAL DIAGNOSIS OF ABNORMALITIES FOUND ON PERIPHERAL SMEAR

I. Basophilic stippling
   A. Lead poisoning
   B. Heavy metal poisoning
   C. Severe anemia
      1. Hemorrhage
      2. Hemolysis
II. Target cells
   A. Hemoglobinopathies
   B. Thalassemia
   C. Iron deficiency
   D. Liver disease
III. Howell-Jolly bodies
   A. Severe hemolytic anemia
   B. Pernicious anemia
   C. Leukemia
   D. Thalassemia
   E. Postsplenectomy

Modified from: Wallach, J.: in *Interpretation of Laboratory Tests*, 3rd Edition, Boston, Little, Brown, & Co., 1978, p. 107.

IV-12 DIFFERENTIAL DIAGNOSIS OF ERYTHROCYTOSIS

I. Erythrocytosis associated with a normal or reduced red cell mass (spurious)
   A. Acute or chronic hemoconcentration (relative)
   B. Spurious polycythemia (also called stress polycythemia or Gaisböck's syndrome)

II. Erythrocytosis associated with an elevated red cell mass (absolute polycythemia)
   A. Polycythemia vera
   B. Secondary polycythemia (increased erythropoietin production)
      1. Systemic hypoxia
         a. High altitude
         b. Cardiac disease with right to left shunt
         c. Chronic pulmonary disease
      2. Decreased blood oxygen carrying capacity, increase in carboxyhemoglobin or methemoglobin
      3. Impaired oxygen delivery, hemoglobin with increased oxygen affinity or congenital decreased red cell 2,3 diphosphoglycerate
      4. Local hypoxia - renal artery stenosis
      5. Autonomous erythropoietin production
         a. Tumors
            1. Hypernephroma
            2. Cerebellar hemangioblastoma
            3. Hepatoma
            4. Uterine fibroids
            5. Pheochromocytoma
            6. Adrenal cortical adenoma
            7. Ovarian carcinoma
         b. Renal disorders
            1. Cysts
            2. Hydronephrosis
            3. Bartter's syndrome
            4. Transplantation
      6. Familial polycythemia due to autonomous erythropoietin production

From Advances in Internal Medicine, vol. 24, p. 260, 1979.

IV-13 CRITERIA FOR THE DIAGNOSIS OF POLYCYTHEMIA VERA

I. Major criteria
   A. Increased red cell mass
   B. Arterial O_2 saturation $\geq 92\%$
   C. Splenomegaly
II. Minor criteria
   A. Thrombocytosis
   B. Leukocytosis
   C. Elevated serum B_{12}

Diagnosis of polycythemia vera is made if patient has all three major criteria *or* first two major criteria and any two minor criteria.

III. Most common presenting symptoms of patients in the national polycythemia vera study

Symptoms	Percentage
Headache	49
Weakness	47
Pruritis	46
Dizziness	45
Sweating	33
Weight loss	31
Paresthesias	29
Joint symptoms	28
Epigastric distress	28

Berlin, N.I.: Diagnosis and classification of polycythemias. Semin. Hematol. 12:339, 1975.

IV-14 CRITERIA FOR THE DIAGNOSIS OF MULTIPLE MYELOMA

I. Major criteria
   A. Plasmacytoma
   B. IgG > 4.0 gm%
      IgA > 2 gm%
      Light chain in urine > 1 gm%
   C. Bone marrow plasma cells > 30%
II. Minor criteria
   A. Bone marrow plasma cells 10-30%
   B. IgG < 4.5
      IgA < 2.0
   C. Lytic bone lesions
   D. Hypogammaglobulinemia

III. To make the diagnosis
   A. I + b, I + c, I + d
   B. II only
   C. III + b, III + c, III + d
   D. a + b + c, a + b + d

Adapted from: Southwest Oncology Group Protocol, 7927.

IV-15 RENAL AND ELECTROLYTE DISORDERS IN MULTIPLE MYELOMA

   I. "Myeloma kidney"
   II. Renal tubular dysfunction
   III. Acute renal failure
   IV. Amyloidosis
   V. Plasma cell invasion of the kidneys
   VI. Hypercalcemia
   VII. Hyperuricemia
   VIII. Spurious hyponatremia
   IX. Urinary tract infections

From: Fer, M.F., et al.: Am. J. Med. 71:707, 1981.

IV-16 CRITERIA FOR THE DIAGNOSIS OF THROMBOTIC THROMBOCYTOPENIC PURPURA

   I. Fever
   II. Microangiopathic hemolytic anemia (Coombs negative)
   III. Thrombocytopenia
   IV. Neurologic disorders
   V. Renal dysfunction

IV-17 DIFFERENTIAL DIAGNOSIS OF SPLENOMEGALY

I. Immunologic-inflammatory
   A. Infections: Subacute bacterial endocarditis, brucellosis, tuberculosis, infectious mononucleosis, cytomegalovirus, syphilis, histoplasmosis, malaria, kala azar schistosomiasis
   B. Connective tissue diseases: rheumatoid arthritis, Felty's syndrome, systemic lupus erythematosus
   C. Sarcoidosis
II. Hematologic disorders
   A. Neoplastic: Lymphomas, histiocytoses, myeloproliferative syndromes (chronic myelocytic leukemia, polycythemia vera, myelofibrosis, and myeloid metaplasia), chronic lymphocytic leukemia, acute leukemia
   B. Nonneoplastic: Hemolytic anemias, e.g., hereditary spherocytosis, autoimmune hemolytic anemia, hemoglobinopathies, immunoblastic lymphadenopathy
III. Congestive splenomegaly due to portal hypertension: Hepatic cirrhosis, portal or splenic vein thrombosis or stenosis, myeloid metaplasia, vinyl chloride
IV. Metabolic-infiltrative: Gaucher's and Niemann-Pick's disease, amyloidosis
V. Miscellaneous: Cyst, splenic abscess, aneurysm of splenic artery, cavernous hemangioma

Adapted from: Fefer, A.: in *Harrison's Principles of Internal Medicine*, Isselbacher, K.J., Adams, R.D., Braunwald, E., Petersdorf, R.G., and Wilson, J.D. (eds.), 9th Edition, McGraw-Hill Book Company, New York City, 1980, p. 282.

IV-18 DIFFERENTIAL DIAGNOSIS OF LYMPHADENOPATHY

I. Neoplastic
  - A. Hematologic: Lymphomas, acute leukemia, chronic lymphocytic leukemia, myeloproliferative syndromes, histiocytoses
  - B. Nonhematologic: Carcinomas of head and neck, lung, breast, kidney

II. Immunologic or inflammatory
  - A. Infections: Pyogenic streptococcal, staphylococcal, and salmonella infections, brucellosis, tuberculosis, syphilis, infectious mononucleosis, cytomegalovirus, infectious hepatitis, rubella, lymphogranuloma venereum, toxoplasmosis, histoplasmosis, coccidioidomycosis, malaria
  - B. Connective tissue diseases: Rheumatoid arthritis, systemic lupus erythematosus, dermatomyositis
  - C. Serum sickness
  - D. Reaction to hydantoins
  - E. Sarcoidosis
  - F. Miscellaneous: Giant (angiofollicular) lymph node hyperplasia, sinus histiocytosis, dermatopathic lymphadenitis, immunoblastic lymphadenopathy

III. Endocrine: Hyperthyroidism, Addison's disease

IV. Lipid storage diseases: Gaucher's and Niemann-Pick's diseases

Adapted from: Fefer, A.: in *Harrison's Principles of Internal Medicine*, Isselbacher, K.J., Adams, R.D., Braunwald, E., Petersdorf, R.G., and Wilson, J.D. (eds.), 9th Edition, McGraw-Hill Book Company, New York City, 1980, p. 280.

IV-19 DIFFERENTIAL DIAGNOSIS OF THROMBOCYTOPENIA

I. Production defect
   A. Reduced thrombopoiesis (reduced megakaryocytes)
      1. Marrow injury: Drugs, chemicals, radiation, infection
      2. Marrow failure: Acquired, congenital (Fanconi's syndrome, amegakaryocytic)
      3. Marrow invasion: Carcinoma, leukemia, lymphoma, fibrosis
      4. Lack of marrow stimulus: Thrombopoietin deficiency
   B. Defective maturation (normal or increased megakaryocytes)
      1. Vitamin B_{12} deficiency, folic acid deficiency
      2. Hereditary: Wiskott-Aldrich syndrome, May-Hegglin anomaly
II. Sequestration (disordered distribution)
   A. Splenomegaly
   B. Hypothermic anesthesia
III. Accelerated destruction
   A. Antibodies
      1. Autoantibodies
         a. ITP, systemic lupus erythematosus, hemolytic anemias, lymphoreticular disorders
         b. Drugs
      2. Alloantibodies
         a. Fetal-maternal incompatibility
         b. Following transfusions
   B. Nonimmunologic
      1. Injury due to:
         a. Infection
         b. Prosthetic heart valves
      2. Consumption
         a. Thrombin in disseminated intravascular coagulation
         b. Thrombotic thrombocytopenic purpura
      3. Loss by hemorrhage and massive transfusion

Adapted from: Nossel, H.L.: in *Harrison's Principles of Internal Medicine*, Isselbacher, K.J., Adams, R.D., Braunwald, E., Petersdorf, R.G., and Wilson, J.D. (eds.), 9th Edition, McGraw-Hill Book Company, New York City, 1980, p. 1555.

IV-20 DIFFERENTIAL DIAGNOSIS OF CYANOSIS

I. Decreased oxygenation of hemoglobin (deoxyhemoglobin)
   A. Reduced arterial oxygen tension (common)
      1. Pulmonary disease
      2. Cardiac right-to-left shunt
   B. Hemoglobin variant having decreased oxygen affinity (rare): Hb Kansas, Hb Beth Israel

II. Methemoglobinemia
   A. Hereditary
   B. Acquired
      1. Nitrites and nitrates: Sodium nitrite, amyl nitrite, nitroglycerin, nitroprusside, silver nitrate
      2. Aniline dyes
      3. Acetanilid and phenacetin
      4. Sulfonamides
      5. Other: Lidocaine, chlorate, phenazopyridine

Modified from: Bunn, H.F.: in *Harrison's Principles of Internal Medicine*, Isselbacher, K.J., Adams, R.D., Braunwald, E., Petersdorf, R.G., and Wilson, J.D. (eds.), 9th Edition, McGraw-Hill Book Company, New York City, 1980, p. 1551.

IV-21 PARANEOPLASTIC SYNDROMES

I. Endocrine
   A. Cushing's syndrome
   B. Hypercalcemia
   C. Gynecomastia
   D. Hypoglycemia
   E. Hypokalemia
   F. S.I.A.D.H.
   G. Carcinoid syndrome
II. Skeletal
   A. Digital clubbing
   B. Hypertrophic pulmonary osteoarthropathy
III. Skin
   A. Dermatomyositis
   B. Acanthosis nigricans
IV. Neurology
   A. Eaton-Lambert syndrome
   B. Peripheral neuropathies
   C. Subacute cerebellar degeneration
   D. Cortical degeneration
   E. Polymyositis
   F. Transverse myelitis
   G. Progressive multifocal leukoencephalopathy
V. Vascular
   A. Thrombophlebitis
   B. Marantic endocarditis
VI. Hematology
   A. Anemia
   B. Dysproteinemia
   C. D.I.C.
   D. Eosinophilia
   E. Leukocytosis
VII. Other
   A. Nephrosis
   B. Hypouricemia

Modified from: Hospital Practice, January 1981

IV-22 CAUSES OF HYPONATREMIA IN CANCER PATIENTS

I. Pseudohyponatremia (multiple myeloma, other paraproteinemias)
II. Adrenal insufficiency
III. Gastrointestinal losses with "pure water" replacement

   A. Tumor-related (usually small cell carcinoma of the lung)
   B. Drug-related (cyclophosphamide, vinca alkaloids, narcotic analgesics, phenothiazines, barbiturates, tricyclic antidepressants)
   C. Infection-related (pulmonary and central nervous system infections)

IV-23 NEOPLASM-RELATED CAUSES OF HYPOKALEMIA

   I. Malignant neoplasms
   A. Colon cancer with diarrhea
   B. Tumors with ectopic ACTH secretion
   C. Adrenal carcinoma
   D. Renal tubular acidosis and Fanconi syndrome secondary to multiple myeloma
   E. Acute myelomonocytic leukemia with lysozymuria
   F. Ectopic renin secretion from renal tumors
   II. "Benign" neoplasms
   A. Pancreatic adenoma with Zollinger-Ellison syndrome
   B. Villous adenoma of the colon
   C. Adrenal adenoma with hyperaldosteronism
   III. Treatment-related
   A. Ureterosigmoidostomy
   B. Laxative overdose
   C. Prolonged corticosteroid therapy

IV-24 FACTORS RELATED TO THE SURVIVAL OF PATIENTS WITH BREAST CANCER

   I. Tumor size
   II. Local skin involvement
   III. Tumor fixation of chest wall
   IV. Presence of palpable axillary nodes
   V. Fixation of axillary nodes
   VI. Presence of supraclavicular nodes
   VII. Generalized inflammation of breast
   VIII. Presence of distant metastasis
   IX. Tumor growth rate

Henderson, I.C. and Canellos, G.P.: Cancer of the Breast: The Past Decade. N. Engl. J. Med. 302:18, 1980.

IV-25 W.H.O. CLASSIFICATION OF MALIGNANT PLEUROPULMONARY NEOPLASMS

   I. Epidermoid carcinomas
  II. Small cell anaplastic carcinoma
 III. Adenocarcinomas
     A. Bronchogenic
     B. Bronchoalveolar
 IV. Large cell carcinomas
  V. Combined epidermoid carcinomas and adenocarcinomas
 VI. Carcinoid tumors
VII. Bronchial gland tumors
     A. Cylindromas
     B. Mucoepidermoid tumors
VIII. Papillary tumors of the surface epithelium
 IX. "Mixed" tumors and carcinosarcomas
  X. Sarcomas
 XI. Unclassified
XII. Melanoma

IV-26 MOST FREQUENT TYPES OF NEOPLASMS IN MALIGNANT PLEURAL EFFUSIONS IN ORDER OF DECREASING INCIDENCE

I. Breast	VI. GI tract
II. Lung	VII. Mesothelioma
III. Lymphoma/leukemia	VIII. Uterus
IV. Ovary	IX. Kidney
V. Unknown primary	X. Sarcoma

Source: Papac, R.J.: in *Cancer: A Comprehensive Treatise*, Frederick F. Becker (Ed.), Plenum Press, New York, 1977, Vol. 5, p. 208.

IV-27 MOST FREQUENT MALIGNANCIES CAUSING PERITONEAL EFFUSIONS (IN ORDER OF DECREASING INCIDENCE)

I. Ovary	V. Breast
II. Stomach	VI. Lymphoma
III. Uterus	VII. Mesothelioma
IV. Unknown primary	

Modified from: Papac, R.J.: in *Cancer: A Comprehensive Treatise*, Frederick F. Becker (Ed.), Plenum Press, New York, 1977, Vol. 5, p. 212.

MOST FREQUENT NEOPLASMS CAUSING MALIGNANT PERICARDIAL EFFUSIONS (IN ORDER OF DECREASING INCIDENCE)
    I. Leukemia, lymphoma
    II. Breast
    III. Lung

Modified from: Papac, R.J.: in *Cancer: A Comprehensive Treatise*, Frederick F. Becker (Ed.), Plenum Press, New York, 1977, Vol. 5, p. 214.

IV-28 HORMONAL BASIS OF HYPERCALCEMIA OF MALIGNANCY
    I. PTH
    II. PTH-like
    III. Osteoclastic activating factor (O.A.F.)
    IV. Prostaglandins
    V. Phosphaturic factor

IV-29 CANCERS MOST LIKELY TO METASTASIZE TO BONE
    I. Thyroid
    II. Breast
    III. Prostate
    IV. Renal
    V. Lung

IV-30 OUTCOME OF TREATMENT OF VARIOUS TUMORS

I. Tumors curable by chemotherapy
   A. Choriocarcinoma
   B. Burkitt's lymphoma
   C. Hodgkin's lymphoma
   D. Acute lymphocytic leukemia - children
   E. Testicular tumors
   F. Wilm's tumor
   G. Ewing's sarcoma
   H. Embryonal rhabdomyosarcoma
   I. Diffuse histocytic lymphoma
II. Tumors in which remissions or increased survival rate are achievable
   A. Acute nonlymphocytic leukemia
   B. Chronic myelocytic leukemia
   C. Chronic lymphocytic leukemia
   D. Multiple myeloma
   E. Non-Hodgkin's lymphoma
   F. "Head and neck" cancer
   G. Adenocarcinoma of the ovary
   H. Small cell anaplastic carcinoma, lung
   I. Soft tissue sarcoma
   J. Neuroblastoma
   K. Adenocarcinoma of colon and rectum
   L. Breast cancer
   M. Malignant melanoma
   N. Islet cell carcinoma
   O. Osteogenic sarcoma
III. Tumors with infrequent response and no increased survival
   A. Brain tumors
   B. GI adenocarcinoma (excluding colon & rectum)
   C. Bronchogenic carcinoma
   D. Cervical and uterine carcinoma
   E. Hypernephroma
   F. Carcinoma of the bladder
   G. Carcinoma of the prostate
   H. "Blast crisis" of chronic myelogenous leukemia
   I. Adrenal carcinoma
   J. Anaplastic thyroid carcinoma
   K. Carcinoid

Kennedy, G.T., et al.: Source: Papac, R.J.: in *Cancer: A Comprehensive Treatise*, Frederick F. Becker (Ed.), Plenum Press, New York, 1977, Vol. 5, p. 18.

IV-31 LONG TERM EFFECTS OF RADIATION

   I. Salivary gland - xerostomia
   II. Esophagus - ulcer, stricture
  III. Stomach - achlorhydria, pyloric stenosis, ulceration
  IV. Small intestine - ulcer, perforation, stricture, malabsorption
   V. Colon - ulcer, perforation, stricture, fistula formation
  VI. Kidney - nephritis
 VII. Bladder - ulceration, contracture, dysuria, frequency
VIII. Lung - pneumonitis, fibrosis
  IX. Heart - pericarditis, pancarditis
   X. Bone - arrested growth - children
  XI. CNS - atrophy
 XII. Spinal cord - transverse myelitis

Cancer: A Comprehensive Treatise, Vol. 5, p. 8, Plenum Press, 1977, Frederick F. Becker, Editor.

IV-32 MYELOTOXICITY FROM CANCER THERAPY

Agent	Nadir of Granulocytes (Days)	Recovery (Days)
Primarily myelosuppressive toxicity		
Ionizing radiations	15	25
Nitrogen mustard	7-15	28
Melphalan	l0-12	
Busulfan	11-30	24-54
BCNU	26-30	35-49
CCNU	40-50	60
Methyl-CCNU	28-63	82-89
Ara-C	12-14	22-24
Vinblastine	5-9	14-21
Myelosuppressive but other complications equally important		
Cyclophosphamide	8-14	18-25
5-Fluorouracil	7-14	
6-Mercaptopurine	7	14-21
Methotrexate	7-14	14-21
Actinomycin D	15	22-25
Procarbazine	25-36	35-50
Myelosuppression not usually the dose limiting toxicity		
Vincristine	4-5	7
Mithramycin	—	—
Streptozotocin	—	—
o.p.' DDD (mitotane)	—	—
Bleomycin	—	—
Rarely if ever cause granulocytopenia		
Prednisone	—	—
Androgens	—	—
Estrogens	—	—
L-Asparaginase	—	—

Adapted from: Henderson. A general guideline. The data vary greatly with the dosage, schedule, and prior forms of the same or concomitant forms of other cancer therapy. Henderson, E.S.: The granulocytopenic effects of cancer chemo- therapeutic agents, in Dimitrov, N.V., and Nodine, J.H. (eds.): Drugs and Hematologic Reactions (New York): Grune & Stratton, New York, 1974, p. 208.

V—Infectious Disease

V-I DISEASE STATES CAUSING FEVER OF UNKNOWN ORIGIN (FUO)*

I. Infection
- A. Generalized
  1. Tuberculosis
  2. Histoplasmosis
  3. Typhoid fever
  4. CMV
  5. EB virus
  6. Miscellaneous: syphilis, brucellosis, toxoplasmosis, malaria
- B. Localized
  1. Infective endocarditis
  2. Empyema
  3. Intraabdominal infection
     a. Peritonitis
     b. Cholangitis
     c. Abscess
  4. Urinary tract
     a. Pyelonephritis
     b. Perinephric abscess
     c. Prostatitis
  5. Decubitus ulcer
  6. Osteomyelitis
  7. Thrombophlebitis

II. Neoplasm
- A. Hematological
  1. Lymphoma
  2. Hodgkin's disease
  3. Acute leukemia
- B. Tumors predisposed to cause fever
  1. Hepatoma
  2. Hypernephroma
  3. Atrial myxoma

III. Connective Tissue Disease
- A. RA, SLE
- B. Vasculitis

IV. Miscellaneous
   A. Drug induced
   B. Immune complex: SLE, RA
   C. Vasculitis
   D. Alcoholic liver disease
   E. Granulomatous hepatitis
   F. Inflammatory bowel disease, Whipple's disease
   G. Recurrent pulmonary emboli
   H. Factitious fever
   I. Undiagnosed

* Diagnostic criteria for FUO

1. Illness of more than three weeks duration
2. Fever, intermittent or continuous
3. Documentation of fever>38.3°C
4. No obvious diagnosis after initial complete examination

V-2 CLASSIFICATION OF TUBERCULOSIS
   I. Tuberculosis exposure, no evidence of infection
  II. Tuberculosis infection, no evidence of disease
      A. Chemotherapy status
 III. Tuberculosis
      A. Location
      B. Bacteriological status
      C. Chemotherapy status

V-3 CLINICAL FEATURES OF GENITOURINARY TUBERCULOSIS

Sterile pyuria	50%
Painless hematuria	40%
Fever	10%
Perinephric abscess	10%
+ sputum culture	20-40%
+ urine culture	80%

Ref: Smith, A.M., Lattimer, J.K.: Genitourinary tract involvement in children with tuberculosis. N.Y. State J. Med. 73:2325, 1973.

V-4 CRITERIA FOR THE DIAGNOSIS OF NONTUBERCULOSIS MYCOBACTERIAL DISEASE

I. The patient should have clinical evidence of disease compatible with the diagnosis

II. Isolation of the organism in colony counts of more than 100 on four or more occasions (with the exception of M. kansasii)

III. Isolation of the organism from ordinarily sterile sources

IV. Culture of the organism from a biopsy specimen

Adapted from: Davidson, PT: The management of disease with atypia mycobacteria. Clin. Notes of Respir., pp. 3-13 (Summer) 1979.

Adapted from: Med. Clinic North Am., vol. 64, No. 3, p. 437, May 1980.

V-5 PULMONARY INFECTIONS IN IMMUNOCOMPROMISED PATIENTS

I. Bacterial
   A. Pseudomonas
   B. Klebsiella
   C. Serratia
   D. Nocardia
   E. Tuberculosis
   F. Listeria
   G. Legionella pneumophilia

II. Fungal
   A. Aspergillus
   B. Candida
   C. Coccidioidomycosis
   D. Cryptococcosis
   E. Phycomycetes

III. Viral
   A. CMV
   B. Herpes simplex
   C. Varicella-zoster
   D. Measles
   E. Adenovirus

IV. Protozoa
   A. Pneumocystis
   B. Toxoplasma

Adapted from: Matthay, RA and Green, WH: Pulmonary Infections in the Immunocompromised patient. Med. Clin. N. Amer. 64:534, 1980.

V-6 CLINICAL PULMONARY SYNDROMES OF HISTOPLASMOSIS

   I. Primary pulmonary histoplasmosis
   II. Histoplasmoma
  III. Fibrosing mediastinitis
  IV. Disseminated histoplasmosis
   V. Chronic cavitary fibronodular pulmonary
  VI. Histoplasmosis

V-7 EXTRAPULMONARY MANIFESTATIONS OF MYCOPLASMA PNEUMONIAE

   I. Hematological
     A. Autoimmune hemolytic anemia
     B. Thrombocytopenia
     C. D.I.C.
     D. Splenomegaly
   II. Gastrointestinal
     A. Gastroenteritis
     B. Anicteric hepatitis
     C. Pancreatitis
  III. Musculoskeletal
     A. Arthralgias
     B. Myalgias
     C. Polyarthritis
  IV. Cardiac
     A. Pericarditis
     B. Myocarditis
     C. Conduction defects
     D. Pericardial effusion
   V. Neurological
     A. Meningitis
     B. Meningoencephalitis
     C. Transverse myelitis
     D. Peripheral and cranial neuropathies
     E. Cerebellar ataxia
  VI. Dermatological
     A. Erythema nodosum
     B. Erythema multiforme
     C. Stevens-Johnson
 VII. Renal
     A. Interstitial nephritis
     B. Glomerulonephritis

Adapted from: Murray, HW and Tuazon, C: Atypical pneumonias. Med Clin N Amer 64:512, 1980.

V-8 EXTRAPULMONARY MANIFESTATIONS OF PSITTACOSIS

I. Cardiac
   A. Myocarditis
   B. Pericarditis
   C. Endocarditis
II. Neurological
   A. Meningitis
   B. Encephalitis
   C. Seizure
III. Hematological
   A. Anemia, non-hemolytic
   B. Hemolytic anemia
   C. D.I.C.
   D. Splenomegaly
IV. Gastrointestinal
   A. Hepatitis
   B. Pancreatitis
V. Renal
   A. Nephritis
   B. Acute renal failure
   C. Proteinuria

Adapted from: Murray, HW, and Tuazon, C: Atypical Pneumonias. Med. Clin. N. Amer. 64:517, 1980.

V-9 EXTRAPULMONARY MANIFESTATIONS OF Q FEVER

I. Gastrointestinal
   A. Hepatitis
II. Cardiovascular
   A. Pericarditis
   B. Myocarditis
   C. Endocarditis
   D. Pericardial effusion
   E. Thrombophlebitis
   F. Arteritis
III. Ocular
   A. Uveitis
   B. Iritis
   C. Optic neuritis
IV. Neurological
   A. Meningitis
   B. Peripheral neuropathy

Adapted from: Murray, HW, and Tuazon, C: Atypical Pneumonias. Med. Clin. N. Amer. 64:521, 1980.

V-10 CLINICAL AND LABORATORY FEATURES OF CYTOMEGALOVIRUS MONONUCLEOSIS*

Clinical	Estimated percent positive
I. Clinical	
A. Prolonged fever (>4 weeks)	20*
B. Hepatomegaly	30-50
C. Splenomegaly	30-50
D. Pharyngitis	5
E. Lymphadenopathy	10
II. Laboratory	
A. Lymphocytosis (>50% of cells)	98
B. Atypical lymphocytes (>20% of lymphocytes)	90
C. Rheumatoid factor, cryoglobulin	30
D. Cold agglutinin (anti-I or anti-i)	25
E. Antinuclear factor	20
F. Coombs' test	10
G. Fourfold CMV CF antibody change	85
H. Virus isolation:	
1. Urine	50-60
2. Saliva	70-90
I. Simultaneous infection with	
1. Epstein-Barr virus	5

*Fever of 2 weeks duration was the criterion for inclusion.

From: Advances in Internal Medicine, Vol. 26, p. 455, 1980.

V-11 FACTORS ASSOCIATED WITH MORTALITY IN BRAIN ABSCESS

   I. Coma on admission
   II. Multiple brain abscesses
   III. Rupture of abscess in ventricle
   IV. Inaccurate or missed diagnosis
   V. Positive spinal fluid cultures
   VI. Brain abscess secondary to remote focus of infection
   VII. Absence of focal signs
 VIII. Seizures
   IX. Symptoms of meningitis early in the illness

Ref: Karandanis, D., Shulman, J.A.: Factors associated with mortality in brain abscess. Arch. Int. Med. 135:1145, 1975.

IV-12 FACTORS AFFECTING MORTALITY OF GRAM-NEGATIVE ROD BACTEREMIA

   I. Absence of fever
   II. Shock
   III. Delayed or inappropriate antibiotic therapy
   IV. Azotemia
   V. Pseudomonas bacteremia
   VI. Severe underlying disease

No association between mortality from gram negative sepsis and age, race, sex, leukocyte count, source of infection was found.

Reference: Bryant, RE, et al.: Arch. Intern. Med. 127:120, 1971.

V-13 OSTEOMYELITIS

I. Microbiology of osteomyelitis
   A. Gram positive cocci (70%)
      1. Staph. aureus
      2. S. epidermidis
      3. S. pyogenes
      4. S. pneumoniae
   B. Gram negative facultative (25%)
      1. Pseudomonas
      2. Serratia
      3. Klebsiella
      4. E. coli
      5. Salmonella
   C. Anaerobic bacteria (2%)
      1. Bacteroides
      2. Peptococci
      3. Peptostreptococci
      4. Fusobacteria
      5. Actinomyces
   D. Other bacteria (1%)
      1. Brucella
      2. Nocardia
   E. Others
      1. M. tuberculosis
      2. Atypical tuberculosis
      3. T. pallidum
      4. Cryptococcus
      5. Coccidioidomycosis
      6. Blastomyces
      7. Candida
      8. Aspergillus
      9. Histoplasma

Ref.: 1. Waldvogel, FA, et al.: N. Engl. J. Med. 1970; 282:198-206, 260-266, 316-322; 302:360-370, 1980.

II. Pathogenesis of osteomyelitis
   A. Hematogenous - 20%
      1. Skin infection
      2. Pneumonia
      3. Urinary tract infection
      4. Gastrointestinal infection
   B. Contiguous focus of infection - 50%
      1. Surgery
      2. Decubitus ulcer
      3. Sinusitis
   C. Peripheral vascular disease - 30%
      1. Diabetes mellitus
      2. Vasculitis

Ref.: Infectious Diseases. Focus on Clinical Diagnosis. H. Thadepalli, M.D., Editor, Medical Examination Publishing Co., Inc., 1980.

V-14 SPECTRUM OF GONOCOCCAL INFECTIONS

I. Urethritis
II. Cervicitis
III. Prostatitis
IV. Epididymitis
V. Pelvic inflammatory disease
VI. Salpingitis
VII. Proctitis
VIII. Conjunctivitis
IX. Pharyngitis
X. Dermatitis
XI. Arthritis
XII. Perihepatitis
XIII. Peritonitis
XIV. Pericarditis
XV. Myocarditis
XVI. Endocarditis
XVII. Hepatitis
XVIII. Meningitis

V-15 CLINICAL FEATURES OF FOOD POISONING SECONDARY TO BOTULISM

I. Visual disturbances (mydriasis, ophthalmoplegia, diplopia)
II. Speech disturbances (dysphonia, dysarthria)
III. Dysphagia
IV. Descending motor paralysis, bilaterally symmetrical
V. Clear sensorium
VI. Fever is unusual
VII. Diarrhea is rare, constipation is the rule

Ref.: Infectious Diseases. Focus on Clinical Diagnosis. H. Thadepalli, M.D., Editor, Medical Examination Publishing Co., Inc. 1980.

V-16 ANTIBIOTIC ASSOCIATED PSEUDOMEMBRANOUS COLITIS

I. Antibiotics implicated

*Lincomycin	Amoxicillin	Erythromycin	Neomycin
*Clindamycin	Cephalosporins	Oral penicillin	Vancomycin
*Ampicillin	Tetracycline	Gentamicin	Sulfa-trimethoprim

II. Clinical features
   A. Diarrhea (rarely bloody)
   B. Crampy abdominal pain and tenderness to palpation
   C. Fever
   D. Toxic megacolon (rare)
   E. Leukocytosis

III. Diagnosis
   A. Pseudomembranous lesion (plaques) visualized at sigmoidoscopy (75-80% of cases)
   B. Demonstration of *C. difficile* toxin

IV. Treatment
   A. Discontinue antibiotics
   B. Vancomycin (metronidazole and bacitracin may also be effective)
      1. 10-15% of patients will relapse after treatment
   C. Bile salt sequestering agents (cholestyramine)

*Especially important

V-17 TOXIC SHOCK SYNDROME

I. Etiology and epidemiology
   A. Approximately 80% of cases occur in women < 30years of age
   B. 10% of cases seen in postmenopausal women and men
      1. Drug abusers
      2. Homosexuals
      3. Patients with staphylococcal sepsis
   C. Strong correlation between toxic shock syndrome and recovery of *S. aureus* from vaginal cultures
   D. Toxins elaborated by *S. aureus* may be responsible for some of the clinical manifestations
II. Clinical features
   A. Multisystem disease
      1. Rash—macular, erythematous, often desquamative
      2. Fever
      3. Hypotension
      4. Volume depletion
      5. Renal insufficiency
      6. Liver test abnormalities
      7. Nausea, vomiting, diarrhea
      8. Thrombocytopenia, subclinical DIC
      9. Disorientation with/without focal neurologic signs
   B. Diagnosis
      1. No. 1-3 and any 3 of items No. 4-9
III. Differential diagnosis
   A. Meningococcemia
   B. Rocky Mountain spotted fever
   C. Leptospirosis
   D. Drug eruptiom
   E. Rubeola

V-18 ACQUIRED IMMUNE DEFICIENCY SYNDROME (AIDS)

I. Etiology and epidemiology
   A. Pathogenesis not yet defined
   B. Occurrence
      1. Homosexuals, mostly males   75-80%
      2. Drug abusers   10-15%
      3. Haitian immigrants   5%
      4. Hemophiliacs   1%
      5. Unclassified   1%

II. Clinical features
   A. Anorexia, malaise, fever, weight loss
   B. Lymphadenopathy, hepatomegaly, splenomegaly
   C. Increased incidence of opportunistic infections
      1. *Pneumocystis carinii*
      2. *Candida albicans*
      3. Cytomegalovirus
      4. Herpes simplex
      5. Mycobacterium avium intracellulare
   D. Increased incidence of Kaposi's sarcoma, Burkitt's lymphoma, non Hodgkin's lymphoma
   E. Lymphopenia
   F. T cell abnormalities
      1. Normal suppressor cell function
      2. Impaired helper cell function
   G. Normal humoral immune function
   H. High fatality rate

VI—Nephrology

VI-1 DIFFERENTIAL DIAGNOSIS OF METABOLIC ALKALOSIS

I. Sodium Chloride-responsive ($U_{Cl^-} < 10$ mmoles per liter)
   A. Gastrointestinal disorders:
      1. Vomiting
      2. Gastric drainage
      3. Villous adenoma of the colon
      4. Chloride diarrhea
   B. Diuretic therapy
   C. Rapid correction of chronic hypercapnia
   D. Cystic fibrosis

II. Sodium Chloride-resistant ($U_{Cl^-} > 20$ mmoles per liter)
   A. Excess mineralocorticoid activity
      1. Hyperaldosteronism
      2. Cushing's syndrome
      3. Bartter's syndrome
      4. Excess licorice intake
   B. Profound potassium depletion

III. Unclassified
   A. Alkali administration
   B. Milk-alkali syndrome
   C. Nonparathyroid hypercalcemia
   D. Massive transfusion
   E. Glucose ingestion after starvation
   F. Large doses of carbenicillin or penicillin

Adapted from: Kaehary, W.D., Gabow, P.A., *Renal & Electrolyte Disorders*, Schrier, R.W. (Ed.), 2nd Edition, Little, Brown and Co., Boston, 1980, p. 146.

VI-2 DIFFERENTIAL DIAGNOSIS OF METABOLIC ACIDOSIS WITH INCREASED ANION GAP

I. Increased Acid Production
  A. Diabetic ketoacidosis
  B. Alcoholic ketoacidosis
  C. Starvation ketoacidosis
  D. Lactic acidosis
      1. Secondary to hypotension, hypovolemia, hypoxemia
      2. Secondary to drugs and toxins
  E. Poisons and drug toxicity
      1. Salicylates
      2. Methanol
      3. Ethylene glycol
      4. Paraldehyde
  F. Hyperosmolar hyperglycemic nonketotic coma
II. Renal Failure
  A. Acute renal failure
  B. Chronic renal failure

Modified from: Levinsky, N.: in *Harrison's Principles of Internal Medicine*, Isselbacher, K.J., Adams, R.D., Braunwald, E., Petersdorf, R.G., and Wilson, J.D. (eds.), 9th Edition, McGraw-Hill Book Company, New York City, 1980, p. 446.

VI-3 DIFFERENTIAL DIAGNOSIS OF METABOLIC ACIDOSIS WITH NORMAL ANION GAP (HYPERCHLOREMIC ACIDOSIS)

I. Renal tubular acidosis
II. Uremic acidosis (early)
III. Intestinal loss of bicarbonate or organic acid anions
  A. Diarrhea
  B. Pancreatic fistula
IV. Ureteroenterostomy
V. Drugs
  A. Acetazolamide
  B. Sulfamylon
  C. Cholestyramine
  D. Acidifying agents: NH_4Cl, oral $Ca\ Cl_2$, arginine-HCl, lysine-HCl
  E. Aldactone (in patients with cirrhosis)
VI. Rapid IV hydration
VII. Connection of respiratory alkalosis
VIII. Hyperalimentation

Modified from: Emmett, M., Narins, R.G.: Clinical use of the anion gap. Medicine 56:38, 1977.

VI-4 DIFFERENTIAL DIAGNOSIS OF A LOW ANION GAP

   I. Reduced concentration of unmeasured anions
      A. Dilution
      B. Hypoalbuminemia
  II. Increased unmeasured cations
      A. Paraproteinemia
      B. Hypercalcemia, hypermagnesemia, tromethane (tris buffer) lithium toxicity
 III. Laboratory error
      A. Systemic error:
         1. Underestimation of serum sodium secondary to severe hypernatremia or hyperviscosity
         2. Bromism
      B. Random error: falsely decreased serum sodium, falsely increased serum chloride or bicarbonate.

Modified from: 1. Oh, Man S., Carroll, Hugh J.: Current concepts. The anion gap. N. Engl. J. Med. 297:814, 1977.

2. Emmett, M., Narrins, R.G.: Clinical use of the anion gap. Medicine 56:38, 1977.

VI-5 DIFFERENTIAL DIAGNOSIS OF HYPOKALEMIA

I. Inadequate dietary intake
II. Gastrointestinal losses
   A. Vomiting
   B. Diarrhea
   C. Chronic laxative abuse
III. Renal losses
   A. Diuretics
   B. Mineralocorticoid excess
      1. Primary aldosteronism
         a. adenoma
         b. bilateral adrenal hyperplasia
      2. Cushing's syndrome
         a. primary adrenal disease
         b. secondary to non-endocrine tumor
      3. Accelerated hypertension
      4. Renal vascular hypertension
      5. Renin producing tumor
      6. Adrenogenital syndrome
      7. Licorice excess
   C. Bartter's syndrome
   D. Liddle's syndrome
   E. Renal tubular acidosis
   F. Metabolic alkalosis
   G. Acute hyperventilation
   H. Starvation
   I. Ureterosigmoidostomy
   J. Antibiotics - carbenicillin, amphotericin, gentamicin
   K. Diabetic ketoacidosis
   L. Acute leukemia
IV. Cellular shift
   A. Alkalosis
   B. Periodic paralysis
   C. Barium poisoning
   D. Insulin administration

Modified from: Kunau, R.T., Stein, J.H., Disorders of Hypo- and Hyperkalemia. Clinical Nephrology 7:173, 1977.

VI-6 DIFFERENTIAL DIAGNOSIS OF HYPERKALEMIA

I. Pseudohyperkalemia
   A. Improper collection of blood
   B. Hematologic disorders with increased white blood cells or platelet counts

II. Exogenous potassium load
   A. Oral or intravenous KCI
   B. Potassium containing drugs
   C. Transfusion
   D. Geophagia

III. Cellular shift of potassium
   A. Tissue damage - trauma, burns, rhabdomyolysis
   B. Destruction of tumor tissue
   C. Digitalis overdose
   D. Acidosis
   E. Hyperkalemic periodic paralysis
   F. Hyperosmolality
   G. Succinylcholine
   H. Arginine infusion

IV. Decreased renal potassium excretion
   A. Acute renal failure
   B. Chronic renal failure
   C. Potassium sparing diuretics
   D. Mineralocorticoid deficiency
      1. Addison's disease
      2. Bilateral adrenalectomy
      3. Hypoaldosteronism
         a. hyporeninemic hypoaldosteronism
         b. heparin therapy
         c. specific enzyme defect
         d. tubular unresponsiveness
   E. Congenital adrenal hyperplasia
   F. Primary defect in potassium transport

Modified from: Kunau, R.T., Stein, J.H.: Disorders of hypo- and hyperkalemia. Clinical Nephrology 7:173, 1977.

VI-7 DIFFERENTIAL DIAGNOSIS OF HYPERNATREMIA

I. Extrarenal water loss
   A. Gastrointestinal
      1. Infantile gastroenteritis (hypertonic dehydration)
      2. Tube feeding in semi-conscious patient - increased osmotic load
      3. Gastrointestinal bleed
   B. Skin
      1. Insensible losses
      2. Burns
      3. Sweat
   C. Lungs - insensible loss
II. Renal water loss
   A. Acute renal failure, diuretic phase
   B. Post obstruction diuresis
   C. Diabetes insipidus
   D. Osmotic diuresis - glycosuria, urea, mannitol
III. Excessive sodium intake (without access to water)
IV. Central nervous system lesions
   A. Impairment of thirst perception
   B. Stuporous or comatose patient
V. Adrenal hyperfunction
   A. Cushing's
   B. Primary hyperaldosteronism

Modified from: Levinsky, N.: in *Harrison's Principles of Internal Medicine*, Isselbacher, K.J., Adams, R.D., Braunwald, E., Petersdorf, R.G., and Wilson, J.D. (eds.), 9th Edition, McGraw-Hill Book Company, New York City, 1980, p. 436.

VI-8 DIFFERENTIAL DIAGNOSIS OF HYPONATREMIA

I. Extracellular fluid - volume depleted
   A. Renal losses
      1. Diuretics
      2. Adrenal insufficiency
      3. Salt losing nephropathy
      4. Renal tubular acidosis with bicarbonaturia
      5. Osmotic diuresis (glucose, mannitol, urea)
   B. Extra-renal losses
      1. Vomiting
      2. Diarrhea
      3. "3rd space" (e.g. burns, pancreatitis, traumatized muscle)

II. Extracellular fluid - normal or modest excess
   A. Hypothyroidism
   B. Syndrome of inappropriate ADH secretion
   C. Pain, emotion, drugs
   D. Glucocorticoid deficiency

III. Extracellular fluid - profound excess (edema)
   A. Nephrotic syndrome
   B. Cirrhosis
   C. Congestive heart failure
   D. Renal failure (acute and chronic)

IV. Artifactual
   A. Laboratory error
   B. Hyperglycemia, hypertriglyceridemia, hyperproteinemia.

Reprinted from Kidney International, Vol. 10, pp. 117-132, 1976. Used by permission.

Modified from: Schrier, R.W., Berl, T.: *Renal and Electrolyte Disorders*. Schrier, R. (Ed.), 2nd Edition, Little, Brown & Co., Boston, 1980, p. 39.

VI-9 DIFFERENTIAL DIAGNOSIS OF RENAL TUBULAR ACIDOSIS (RTA) TYPE I (DISTAL)

I. Primary
   A. Sporadic
   B. Genetic

II. Genetically transmitted systemic diseases
   A. Marfan's syndrome
   B. Sickle cell anemia
   C. Carbonic anhydrase B deficiency
   D. Galactosemia
   E. Hereditary fructose intolerance
   F. Ehler's-Danlos syndrome
   G. Fabry's disease
   H. Hereditary elliptocytosis

III. Metabolic disorders
    A. Idiopathic hypercalciuria - sporadic and hereditary
    B. Hyperthyroidism
    C. Primary hyperparathyroidisim
    D. Vitamin D intoxication
    E. Mineralocorticoid deficiency
IV. Hypergammaglobulinemic disorders
    A. Amyloidosis
    B. Idiopathic hyperglobulinemia
    C. Hyperglobulinemic purpura
    D. Cryoglobulinemia
V. Medullary sponge kidney
VI. Hepatic cirrhosis
VII. Wilson's disease
VIII. Drug induced
    A. Amphotericin B
    B. Vitamin D
    C. Lithium
    D. Toluene
    E. Cyclamate
    F. Analgesics
    G. Amiloride
    H. Digoxin (?)
IX. Pyelonephritis
X. Leprosy
XI. Renal transplantation
XII. Obstructive nephropathy
XIII. Autoimmune disorders
    A. Sjögren's syndrome
    B. Thyroiditis
    C. Fibrosing alveolitis
    D. Primary biliary cirrhosis
    E. Systemic lupus erythematosus
    F. Lipoid hepatitis
XIV. Multiple myeloma
XV. Hodgkin's disease

Modified from: Sebastian, A., McSherry, E., Morris, R.: *The Kidney*; Brenner, B., and Rector, F. (Eds.), Vol. I, W.B. Saunders Co., Philadelphia, 1976, p. 623.

VI-10 DIFFERENTIAL DIAGNOSIS OF RENAL TUBULAR ACIDOSIS (RTA) TYPE II (PROXIMAL)

I. Primary
   A. Sporadic
   B. Genetic-Fanconi's syndrome
II. Inborn errors of metabolism
   A. Wilson's disease
   B. Cystinosis
   C. Others: Tyrosinosis, Lowe's syndrome, hereditary fructose intolerance, pyruvate carboxylase deficiency, galactosemia, glycogen storage disease (Type II)
III. Metabolic disorders
   A. Vitamin D deficiency
   B. Primary or secondary hyperparathyroidism
   C. Pseudo-vitamin D-deficiency
IV. Disorders of protein metabolism
   A. Nephrotic syndrome
   B. Multiple myeloma
   C. Sjögren's syndrome
   D. Amyloidosis
   E. Other dysproteinemias
V. Medullary cystic disease
VI. Renal transplantation
VII. Drugs: outdated tetracycline, 6-mercaptopurine, streptozotocin, toluene, sulfonamide, sulfamylon, acetazolamide
VIII. Heavy metals: lead, cadmium, mercury

VI-11 DIFFERENTIAL DIAGNOSIS OF RENAL TUBULAR ACIDOSIS (RTA) TYPE IV

I. Aldosterone deficiency
   A. Combined deficiency of aldosterone and adrenal glucocorticoid hormones
      1. Addison's disease
      2. Bilateral adrenalectomy
      3. Inherited impairment of steroidogenesis: 21-hydroxylase deficiency ("congenital adrenal hyperplasia")
   B. Selective deficiency of aldosterone
      1. Inherited impairment of aldosterone biosynthesis: corticosterone methyl oxidase deficiency
      2. Secondary to deficient renin secretion
         a. Diabetic nephropathy
         b. Chronic tubulo-interstitial disease with glomerular insufficiency
         c. Indomethacin administration
      3. Chronic idiopathic hypoaldosteronism in adults and children

II. Pseudohypoaldosteronism (attenuated renal response to aldosterone with secondary hyperreninemia and hyperaldosteronism)
   A. Classic pseudohypoaldosteronism of infancy
   B. Chronic tubulo-interstitial disease with glomerular insufficiency "salt-wasting nephritis"
   C. Drugs: spironolactone; amiloride; triamterene

III. Attenuated renal response to aldosterone + aldosterone deficiency
   A. Selective tubule dysfunction with impaired renin secretion
   B. Chronic tubulo-interstitial disease with glomerular insufficiency
      1. Associated deficient renin secretion
      2. Renin status uncertain
   C. Renal transplantation with deficient renin secretion
   D. Lupus nephritis with deficient renin secretion

IV. Uncertain pathophysiology
   A. Chronic pyelonephritis
   B. Lupus nephritis
   C. Renal transplantation
   D. Acute glomerulonephritis
   E. Renal amyloidosis

References: Sebastian, et al.: Am. J. Med. 72:301, 1982.

VI-12 DIFFERENTIAL DIAGNOSIS OF PARENCHYMAL RENAL DISEASES CAUSING ACUTE RENAL FAILURE

I. Acute glomerulonephritis
   A. Acute poststreptococcal glomerulonephritis
   B. Systemic lupus erythematosus
   C. Bacterial endocarditis
   D. Goodpasture's syndrome
   E. Schönlein-Henoch purpura
   F. Hypersensitivity angiitis
II. Bilateral cortical necrosis
   A. Obstetrical accidents
   B. Gram negative septicemia
   C. Ischemia
   D. Hyperacute allograft resection
   E. Gastroenteritis (children)
III. Bilateral papillary necrosis
   A. Analgesic abuse
   B. Sickle cell disease
   C. Diabetes mellitus
IV. Diseases of tubules and/or interstitium
   A. Acute pyelonephritis
   B. Acute allergic interstitial nephritis
   C. Hypokalemic nephropathy
   D. Hypercalcemia
   E. Acute uric acid nephropathy
   F. Myeloma of the kidney
V. Diseases of the renal vasculature
   A. Renal artery occlusion
   B. Renal vein thrombosis
   C. Accelerated hypertension
   D. Accelerated scleroderma
VI. Acute nephrotoxic and/or postischemic renal failure

Modified from: Finn, W.F.: in *Strauss and Welt's Diseases of the Kidney*, Earley, L.E., Gottschalk, C.W. (eds.), Boston, 3rd Edition, Little, Brown and Co., 1979, p. 168.

VI-13 DIFFERENTIAL DIAGNOSIS OF ACUTE DETERIORATION IN RENAL FUNCTION

    I. Prerenal failure
- A. Hypovolemia
- B. Cardiovascular failure

   II. Postrenal failure
- A. Obstruction
- B. Bladder rupture

  III. Acute reversible renal failure (acute tubular necrosis)
- A. Postischemia
- B. Pigment induced
  1. Hemolysis
  2. Rhabdomyolysis
- C. Toxin induced
  1. Antibiotics
  2. Contrast material
  3. Anesthetic agents
  4. Heavy metals
  5. Organic solvents
- D. Intratubular precipitation
  1. Uric acid
  2. Oxalate
- E. Hypercalcemia
- F. Diffuse pyelonephritis

Modified from: Anderson, R., Schrier, R.: in *Harrison's Principles of Internal Medicine*, Isselbacher, K.J., Adams, R.D., Braunwald, E., Petersdorf, R.G., and Wilson, J.D. (eds.), 9th Edition, McGraw-Hill Book Company, New York City, 1980, p. 1293.

VI-14 DIFFERENTIAL DIAGNOSIS OF COMMON MECHANICAL CAUSES OF URINARY TRACT OBSTRUCTION

Ureter*	Bladder outlet†	Urethra†
CONGENITAL		
Ureteropelvic junction narrowing or obstruction	Bladder neck obstruction	Posterior urethral valves
Ureterovesical junction narrowing or obstruction	Ureterocele	Anterior urethral valves
Ureterocele		Stricture
Retrocaval ureter		Meatal stenosis
		Phimosis
ACQUIRED INTRINSIC DEFECTS		
Calculi	Benign prostatic hypertrophy	Stricture
Inflammation	Cancer of prostate	Tumor
Trauma	Cancer of bladder	Calculi
Sloughed papillae	Calculi	Trauma
Tumor	Diabetic neuropathy	Phimosis
Blood clots	Spinal cord disease	
Uric acid crystals		
ACQUIRED EXTRINSIC DEFECTS		
Pregnant uterus	Carcinoma of cervix, colon	Trauma
Retroperitoneal fibrosis		
Aortic aneurysm		
Uterine leiomyomata		
Carcinoma of uterus, prostate, bladder, colon, rectum		
Retroperitoneal lymphoma		
Accidental surgical ligation		

* Lesions are typically associated with unilateral obstruction.
† Lesions are typically associated with bilateral obstruction.

Adapted from: Brenner, B., Humes, H.: in *Harrison's Principles of Internal Medicine*, Isselbacher, K.J., Adams, R.D., Braunwald, E., Petersdorf, R.G., and Wilson, J.D. (eds.), 9th Edition, McGraw-Hill Book Company, New York City, 1980, p. 1353.

VI-15 MAJOR NEPHROTOXINS

I. Exogenous
- A. Metals (Hg, Au, Ag, Ar, Pb, Cd, Ur, Li)
- B. Solvents (halogenated hydrocarbons)
- C. Diagnostic agents (contrast agents)
- D. Therapeutic agents
  1. Antibiotics (aminoglycosides, amphotericin B, sulfa's)
  2. Analgesics (phenacetin, ASA)
  3. Anesthetics (methoxyflurane)
  4. Hormones (vitamin D)
  5. Antineoplastics (methotrexate, cis-platinum, cyclophos)
  6. Radiation
- E. Miscellaneous (venoms, mushrooms, fluoride)

II. Endogenous
- A. Uric acid
- B. Oxalate
- C. Pigments (myoglobin, hemoglobin)
- D. Light chain disease
- E. Hormones (PTH)

VI-16 DIFFERENTIATION OF DEHYDRATION AND ACUTE TUBULAR INJURY AS A CAUSE OF OLIGURIA

	U_{osm}	U_{Na} mEq	U/P creatinine	Renal failure index $\dfrac{U_{Na}}{U/P\ creatinine}$	Fractional Excretion Na. $\left[\dfrac{U/P\ Na}{U/P\ creatinine} \times 100\right]$	Hippuran scan	Response to fluid challenge with increased urine output
Dehydration	>300	<20	>14:1	<1	<1	Kidneys well visualized	(+)
Acute tubular necrosis	300	>30	<14:1	>1	>1	Kidney poorly visualized or not at all	(−)

VI-17 DIFFERENTIAL DIAGNOSIS OF ACUTE GLOMERULONEPHRITIS

I. Infectious diseases
   A. Poststreptococcal glomerulonephritis
   B. Nonpoststreptococcal glomerulonephritis
      1. Bacterial: Infective endocarditis, "shunt nephritis," sepsis, pneumococcal pneumonia, typhoid fever, secondary syphilis, meningococcemia
      2. Viral: Hepatitis B, infectious mononucleosis, mumps, measles, varicella, vaccinia, echovirus, and coxsackievirus
      3. Parasitic: Malaria, toxoplasmosis
II. Multisystem diseases: Systemic lupus erythematosus, vasculitis, Schönlein-Henoch purpura, Goodpasture's syndrome
III. Primary glomerular diseases: Membranoproliferative glomerulonephritis, Berger's disease, "pure" mesangial proliferative glomerulonephritis
IV. Miscellaneous: Guillain-Barré syndrome, irradiation of Wilms' tumor, self-administered diphtheria-pertussis-tetanus vaccine, serum sickness

Adapted from: Glasslock, R., Brenner, R.: in *Harrison's Principles of Internal Medicine*, Isselbacher, K.J., Adams, R.D., Braunwald, E., Petersdorf, R.G., and Wilson, J.D. (eds.), 9th Edition, McGraw-Hill Book Company, New York City, 1980, p. 1311.

VI-18 DIFFERENTIAL DIAGNOSIS OF THE NEPHROTIC SYNDROME

I. Primary glomerular disease
  A. Minimal change disease
  B. Focal and segmental glomerulosclerosis
  C. Membranous glomerulonephropathy
  D. Proliferative glomerulonephritis
II. Secondary to other diseases
  A. Infections
    1. Poststreptococcal glomerulonephritis
    2. Endocarditis
    3. Hepatitis B
    4. Syphilis
  B. Drugs and toxins
    1. Anticonvulsants
    2. Penicillamine
  C. Neoplasms
  D. Multisystem disease
    1. Systemic lupus erythematosus
    2. Goodpasture's syndrome
    3. Dermatitis herpetiformis
    4. Amyloidosis
    5. Sarcoidosis
    6. Dermatomyositis
    7. Sjögren's syndrome
  E. Heredo Familial
    1. Diabetes mellitus
    2. Familial or congenital nephrotic syndrome
    3. Sickle cell disease
  F. Miscellaneous
    1. Myxedema
    2. Allergens (bee stings, poisoning, serum sickness)
    3. Renovascular hypertension
    4. Chronic allograft rejection

Modified from: Glassock, R., Brenner, B.: in *Harrison's Principles of Internal Medicine*, Isselbacher, K.J., Adams, R.D., Braunwald, E., Petersdorf, R.G., and Wilson, J.D. (eds.), 9th Edition, McGraw-Hill Book Company, New York City, 1980, p. 1316.

VI-19 DIFFERENTIAL DIAGNOSIS OF TUBULOINTERSTITIAL DISEASE OF THE KIDNEY

I. Toxins
  A. Exogenous toxins
    1. Analgesic nephropathy
    2. Lead nephropathy
    3. Miscellaneous nephrotoxins (e.g., antibiotics, radiographic contrast media, heavy metals)
  B. Metabolic toxins
    1. Acute uric acid nephropathy
    2. Gouty nephropathy
    3. Hypercalcemic nephropathy
    4. Hypokalemic nephropathy
    5. Miscellaneous metabolic toxins (e.g., hyperoxaluria, cystinosis, Fabry's disease)
II. Neoplasia
  A. Lymphoma
  B. Leukemia
  C. Multiple myeloma
III. Immune disorders
  A. Hypersensitivity nephropathy
  B. Sjögren's syndrome
  C. Amyloidosis (see also Chap. 64)
  D. Transplant rejection (see Chap. 69)
  E. Tubulointerstitial abnormalities associated with glomerulonephritis (see also Chaps. 278 and 279)
IV. Vascular disorders (see Chaps. 275 and 282)
  A. Arteriolar nephrosclerosis
  B. Atheroembolic disease
  C. Sickle-cell nephropathy
  D. Acute tubular necrosis
V. Hereditary renal disease
  A. Hereditary nephritis (Alport's syndrome) (see Chap. 279)
  B. Medullary cystic disease (see Chap. 283)
  C. Medullary sponge kidney (see Chap. 283)
VI. Infectious injury (see Chap. 280)
  A. Acute pyelonephritis
  B. Chronic pyelonephritis
VII. Miscellaneous disorders
  A. Chronic urinary tract obstruction (see Chap. 285)
  B. Radiation nephritis
  C. Balkan nephropathy

Adapted from: Brenner, B., Hosteter, T., Humos, H.: in *Harrison's Principles of Internal Medicine*, Isselbacher, K.J., Adams, R.D., Braunwald, E., Petersdorf, R.G., and Wilson, J.D. (eds.), 9th Edition, McGraw-Hill Book Company, New York City, 1980, p. 1334.

VI-20 DIFFERENTIAL DIAGNOSIS OF NEPHROGENIC DIABETES INSIPIDUS

   I. Congenital/familial
  II. Renal disease
     A. Post-obstructive uropathy
     B. Unilateral renal artery stenosis
     C. Renal transplantation
     D. Acute tubular necrosis
 III. Primary hyperaldosteronism
     A. Other causes of hypokalemia
 IV. Hyperparathyroidism
     A. Other causes of hypercalcemia
  V. Drugs
     A. Methoxyflurane anesthesia
     B. Lithium
     C. Demeclocycline
 VI. Systemic diseases
     A. Multiple myeloma
     B. Amyloidosis
     C. Sickle-cell anemia
     D. Sjögren's syndrome

Modified from: Streeten, D., Moses, A., Miller, M.: in *Harrison's Principles of Internal Medicine*, Isselbacher, K.J., Adams, R.D., Braunwald, E., Petersdorf, R.G., and Wilson, J.D. (eds.), 9th Edition, McGraw-Hill Book Company, New York City, 1980, p. 1690.

VI-21 DIFFERENTIAL DIAGNOSIS OF CENTRAL DIABETES INSIPIDUS

   I. Idiopathic
      A. Sporadic
      B. Familial
  II. Head trauma
 III. Neurosurgical procedures
  IV. Neoplasms
      A. Craniopharyngioma
      B. Pinealoma
      C. Metastatic (e.g. breast cancer)
   V. Lymphoma/leukemia
  VI. Infection and granulomatous disease
      A. Encephalitis
      B. Meningitis
      C. Tuberculosis
      D. Syphilis
      E. Sarcoidosis
      F. Eosinophilic granuloma
 VII. Vascular accidents
      A. Thrombosis
      B. Hemorrhage
      C. Sheehan's syndrome
VIII. Histiocytosis

Modified from: Oliver, R., Jamison, R.: Diabetes Insipidus: A Physiologic Approach. Postgraduate Medicine 68:120, 1980.

VI-22 DIFFERENTIAL DIAGNOSIS OF HYPERURICEMIA

  I. Overproduction of uric acid
- A. Primary gout
- B. Myeloproliferative disorders
- C. Lymphoma
- D. Hemoglobinopathies
- E. Hemolytic anemia
- F. Psoriasis
- G. Cancer chemotherapy

 II. Underexcretion of uric acid
- A. Chronic renal failure
- B. Lead nephropathy (saturnine gout)
- C. Drugs (diuretics except spironolactone and ticrynafen; ethambutol; low-dose aspirin)
- D. Lactic acidosis (alcoholism, preeclampsia)
- E. Ketosis (diabetic, starvation)
- F. Hyperparathyroidism
- G. Hypertension

III. Overproduction and underexcretion
    Glycogen storage disease, Type I

IV. Mechanism unknown
- A. Sarcoidosis
- B. Obesity
- C. Hypoparathyroidism
- D. Paget's disease
- E. Down's syndrome

Adapted from: Beary, J.: Manual of Rheumatology and Outpatient Orthopedics. Little, Brown & Co., Boston, 1981, p. 146.

VI-23 DIFFERENTIAL DIAGNOSIS OF NEPHROLITHIASIS

I. Calcium stones
    A. Idiopathic hypercalciuria
    B. Hyperuricosuria
    C. Primary hyperparathyroidism
    D. Distal renal tubular acidosis (RTA)
    E. Hyperoxaluria
        1. Intestinal hyperoxaluria
        2. Hereditary
    F. Idiopathic stone disease
II. Uric acid stones
    A. Gout
    B. Idiopathic
    C. Dehydration
    D. Lesch-Nyhan syndrome
    E. Neoplasm
III. Cystine stones (hereditary)
IV. Struvite stones (infection)

Modified from: Coe, F., Favus, M.: in *Harrison's Principles of Internal Medicine*, Isselbacher, K.J., Adams, R.D., Braunwald, E., Petersdorf, R.G., and Wilson, J.D. (eds.), 9th Edition, McGraw-Hill Book Company, New York City, 1980, p. 1350.

—

VI-24 DIFFERENTIAL DIAGNOSIS OF HYPOURICEMIA

I. Decreased production
   A. Congenital xanthine oxidase deficiency
   B. Liver disease
   C. Allopurinol administration
   D. Low PP-ribose-P synthetase activity
II. Increased excretion
   A. "Isolated" defect in renal transport of uric acid
      1. Idiopathic
      2. Neoplastic diseases
      3. Liver disease
   B. Generalized defect in renal tubular transport (Fanconi's syndrome)
      1. Idiopathic
      2. Wilson's disease
      3. Cystinosis
      4. Multiple myeloma
      5. Heavy metals
      6. Type I glycogen storage disease
      7. Galactosemia
      8. Hereditary fructose intolerance
      9. Outdated tetracyclines
      10. Bronchogenic carcinoma and other neoplasms
      11. Liver disease and alcoholism
   C. Drugs
      1. Acetoheximide
      2. Azauridine
      3. Benzbromarone
      4. Benziodarone
      5. Calcium ipodate
      6. Chlorprothixene
      7. Cinchophen
      8. Citrate
      9. Dicumarol
      10. Diflumidone
      11. Estrogens
      12. Ethyl biscoumacetate
      13. Ethyl p-chlorophenoxyisobutyric acid
      14. Glyceryl guaiacolate
      15. Glycine
      16. Glycopyrrolate
      17. Halofenate
      18. Iodopyracet
      19. Iopanoic acid
      20. Meglumine iodipamide
      21. p-Nitrophenylbutazone
      22. Orotic acid

III. Mechanism unknown
    A. Pernicious anemia
    B. Acute intermittent porphyria

Adapted from: Wyngaarden, J., Kelley, Wm.: in *Gout and Urate Metabolism*, Grune & Stratton, New York, 1976, p. 412.

VI-25 RENAL COMPLICATIONS OF NEOPLASMS

  I. Glomerulonephritis, with or without nephrotic syndrome
 II. Obstructive uropathy
    A. Tubular precipitation syndromes
      1. Uric acid nephropathy
      2. Hypercalcemic nephropathy
      3. Paraproteinuric syndromes
        a. multiple myeloma
        b. other (monoclonal gammopathy, lysozymuria, mucoproteins, proteolytic products)
    B. Obstruction of the ureters, bladder and urethra
III. Direct invasion by malignant process
    A. Primary renal tumors
    B. Metastatic infiltration
IV. Treatment-related nephropathies
    A. Radiation nephropathy
    B. Drug-induced nephrotoxicity
      1. Cytotoxic drugs
      2. Drugs used in supportive care
        a. antibiotics
        b. analgesics
      3. Immunotherapy
 V. Miscellaneous
    A. Disseminated intravascular coagulation
    B. Amyloidosis
    C. Electrolyte abnormalities

Taken from: Fer, et al.: Amer. J. Med. 71:705, 1981

VII—Pulmonary Disease

VII-1 DIFFERENTIAL DIAGNOSIS OF CLUBBING OF THE DIGITS

I. Pulmonary disorders
    A. Infection
        1. Bronchiectasis
        2. Lung abscess
        3. Empyema
        4. Tuberculosis (only with extensive fibrosis or abscess)
    B. Neoplasm
        1. Primary lung cancer
        2. Metastatic lung cancer
        3. Mesothelioma
    C. Pulmonary fibrosis
    D. Arteriovenous malformations
    E. Neurogenic diaphragmatic tumors
II. Cardiac disorders
    A. Congenital cyanotic heart disease
    B. Infective endocarditis
III. Gastrointestinal disorders
    A. Ulcerative colitis
    B. Regional enteritis
IV. Cerebrovascular accident (associated with hemiplegia)
V. Congenital

Modified from: Lanken, P.N. and Fishman, A.P.: in *Pulmonary Diseases and Disorders*, Fishman, A.P. (ed.), Vol. 1, McGraw-Hill Book Company, New York, 1980, p. 87.

VII-2 DIFFERENTIAL DIAGNOSIS OF HEMOPTYSIS

  I. Infections
     *A. Bronchitis, esp. chronic
      B. Bronchiectasis
     *C. Pneumonia
      D. Lung abscess
      E. Tuberculosis
      F. Fungal
 II. Neoplasms
     *A. Bronchogenic adenoma
      B. Bronchial adenoma
III. Cardiovascular disorders
     *A. Pulmonary infarction
      B. Mitral stenosis
      C. Pulmonary congestion and alveolar edema
      D. Aortic aneurysm
      E. Pulmonary arteriovenous fistula
 IV. Trauma
  V. Miscellaneous
      A. Foreign body
      B. Broncholith
      C. Bleeding diathesis
      D. Goodpasture's syndrome
      E. Idiopathic hemosiderosis

* Most common

Modified from: Fishman, A.P.: in *Pulmonary Diseases and Disorders*, Fishman, A.P. (ed.), Vol. 1, McGraw-Hill Book Company, New York, 1980, p. 74.

VII-3 DIFFERENTIAL DIAGNOSIS OF RIB NOTCHING ON CHEST X-RAY

I. Erosions of inferior rib margins
  A. Aortic obstruction
    1. Coarctation of aortic arch
    2. Thrombosis of abdominal aorta
  B. Subclavian artery obstruction
    1. Blalock-Taussig operation
    2. "Pulseless disease"
  C. Tetralogy of Fallot
  D. Pulmonary atresia
  E. Ebstein's malformation
  F. Pulmonary valve stenosis
  G. Unilateral absence of the pulmonary artery
  H. Pulmonary emphysema
  I. Superior vena cava obstruction
  J. Arteriovenous fistula
  K. Intercostal neuroma
  L. Hyperparathyroidism
  M. Idicpathic
  N. Normal
II. Erosions of superior rib margins
  A. Paralytic poliomyelitis
  B. Connective tissue diseases
    1. Rheumatoid arthritis
    2. Scleroderma
    3. SLE
    4. Sjögren's
  C. Localized pressure
    1. Rib retractors
    2. Chest tubes
    3. Multiple hereditary exostosis
    4. Neurofibromatosis
    5. Thoracic neuroblastoma
    6. Coarctation of the aorta
  D. Osteogenesis imperfecta
  E. Marfan's syndrome
  F. Radiation damage
  G. Hyperparathyroidism
  H. Idiopathic

Adapted from: Fraser, R.G.; Pare, J.A.: *Diagnosis of Diseases of the Chest*, 2nd ed., Vol. III, Saunders Co., Philadelphia, 1979, pp. 1892-1895.

VII-4 DIFFERENTIAL DIAGNOSIS OF PLEURAL EFFUSIONS

I. Transudates
   A. Congestive heart failure
   B. Nephrotic syndrome
   C. Superior vena cava obstruction
   D. Liver conditions with ascites (hepatic hydrothorax)
   E. Peritoneal dialysis

II. Exudates
   A. Parapneumonic effusions (viral, bacterial, fungal)
   B. Pulmonary infarction
   C. Collagen vascular disease
      1. Rheumatoid arthritis
      2. Systemic lupus erythematosus
   D. Neoplasms
   E. Subphrenic inflammatory conditions
   F. Hypoplasia or obstruction of lymphatics
   G. Pancreatitis

III. Hemorrhagic
   A. Trauma
   B. Pulmonary infarction
   C. Neoplasms
   D. Tuberculosis

IV. Lipidic
   A. Chylous
      1. Rupture of thoracic duct
      2. Rupture or obstruction of other lymphatics (cysterna chyli)
   B. Cholesterol - any long standing cellular effusion

V. Empyema

Modified from: Johnston, R.F., et al.: in *Pulmonary Diseases and Disorders*, Fishman, A.P. (ed.), Vol. 2, McGraw-Hill Book Company, New York, 1980, p. 1366.

VII-5 CRITERIA FOR TRANSUDATIVE AND EXUDATIVE EFFUSIONS

	Transudate	Exudate
Pleural fluid protein g/dl	< 3.0	> 3.0
$\dfrac{\text{Pleural fluid total protein}}{\text{Serum fluid total protein}}$	< 0.5	> 0.5
$\dfrac{\text{Pleural fluid LDH}}{\text{Serum LDH}}$	< 0.6	> 0.6
Pleural fluid specific gravity	< 1.016	> 1.0.6

Light, R.W., MacGregor, M.L., Luchsinger, P.D., Ball, W.C.: Pleural effusions: The diagnostic separation of transudates and exudates. Ann. Int. Med. 77:507-513, 1972.

VII-6 DIFFERENTIAL DIAGNOSIS OF COUGH WITH NEGATIVE CHEST X-RAY

    I. Acute respiratory infections
    II. Acute irritative bronchitis (inhaled or aspirated irritant)
    III. Postbronchitis cough syndrome
    IV. Chronic bronchitis
    V. Asthma
    VI. Bronchiectasis
    VII. Congestive heart failure
    VIII. Esophageal disease which result in recurrent aspiration
        A. Esophageal reflux
        B. Achalasia
        C. Zenker's diverticulum
    IX. Tracheobronchial neoplasms
        A. Primary tracheal tumors
        B. Secondary tracheal malignancy
        C. Bronchogenic carcinoma
        D. Bronchial adenoma
        E. Metastatic tumors
    X. Non-neoplastic bronchial obstructive lesions
        A. Foreign body
        B. Broncholithiasis
        C. Bronchial stricture
        D. Extrinsic compression
    XI. Cystic fiber
    XII. Laryngeal lesions
    XIII. Post nasal discharge
    XIV. Psychogenic cough

VII-7 DIFFERENTIAL DIAGNOSIS OF UNILATERAL HILAR ENLARGEMENT

I. Malignancy
   A. Primary bronchogenic carcinoma
   B. Metastatic lymphadenopathy
II. Infections
   A. TB
   B. Fungal
   C. Bacterial (occasionally)
III. Sarcoidosis
IV. Lymph node hyperplasia
V. Pulmonary artery enlargement
VI. Mediastinal masses

VII-8 DIFFERENTIAL DIAGNOSIS OF BILATERAL HILAR ENLARGEMENT

I. Sarcoidosis
II. Infection
   A. Tuberculosis
   B. Fungal
   C. Mononucleosis
   D. Mycoplasma
III. Metastatic tumor
IV. Lymphoma
V. Pneumoconioses
   A. Silicosis
   B. Berylliosis
   C. Bauxite fibrosis
VI. Vascular
   A. Enlargement of pulmonary arteries
      1. Pulmonary emboli, recurrent (or massive)
      2. Chronic cor pulmonale
   B. Enlargement of pulmonary veins
      1. Congestive heart failure
      2. Mitral stenosis

VII-9 DIFFERENTIAL DIAGNOSIS OF PNEUMOTHORAX

I. Primary spontaneous pneumothorax
II. Iatrogenic
III. Traumatic
IV. Mediastinal emphysema
V. Pulmonary inflammation
    A. Tuberculosis
    B. Coccidioidomycosis (other fungal infections less commonly)
    C. Staphylococcal pneumonia with abscess (other bacterial pneumonias)
VI. Rupture of cysts and bullae
VII. "Honeycomb" lungs (pulmonary microcysts)
    A. Idiopathic
    B. Cystic fibrosis
    C. Scleroderma
    D. Eosinophilic granuloma
    E. Pulmonary tuberous sclerosis
    F. Pulmonary lymphangiomatoid granulomatosis
    G. Pneumoconioses
    H. Marfan's syndrome
VIII. Catamenial pneumothorax
IX. Miscellaneous
    A. Primary or secondary
    B. Pulmonary infarction with cavitation
    C. Sarcoidosis

VII-10 DIFFERENTIAL DIAGNOSIS OF RECURRENT PULMONARY INFECTION ASSOCIATED WITH IMMUNODEFICIENCY SYNDROMES

I. Antibody (B-cell) deficiency syndromes
   A. Common, variable, acquired hypogammaglobulinemia
   B. Congenital, X-linked hypogammaglobulinemia
   C. Transient hypogammaglobulinemia of infancy
   D. Selective IgA deficiency
   E. Selective IgM deficiency
   F. Selective IgG subclass deficiency
II. Complement deficiency syndromes
   A. C'3 deficiency
   B. C'5 dysfunction
III. Phagocyte deficiency syndromes
   A. Granulocytopenia
   B. Chronic granulomatous disease
   C. Myeloperoxidase deficiency
   D. Chediak-Higashi syndrome
   E. "Lazy leukocyte" syndrome
IV. Cellular (T-cell) deficiency syndromes
   A. Congenital thymic aplasia
   B. Chronic mucocutaneous candidiasis
V. Combined antibody and cellular deficiency syndromes
   A. Severe combined immunodeficiency
   B. Ataxia-telangiectasia
   C. Wiskott-Aldrich syndrome

Modified from: Daubek, J.H., et al.: in *Pulmonary Diseases and Disorders*, Fishman, A.P. (ed.), Vol. 2, McGraw-Hill Book Company, New York, 1980, p. 1002.

VII-11 DIFFERENTIAL DIAGNOSIS OF EOSINOPHILIC LUNG DISEASE

I. Idiopathic
 A. Transient pulmonary eosinophilia (Loeffler's)
 B. Prolonged pulmonary eosinophilia (Carrington's)
II. Eosinophilic lung disease of specific etiology
 A. Drug induced (i.e. nitrofurantoin)
 B. Parasite induced
  1. Strongyloides
  2. Ancylostomiasis
  3. Tropical pulmonary eosinophilia
  4. Pulmonary larva nigrans
  5. Schistosomiasis
 C. Fungus induced
  1. Hypersensitivity bronchopulmonary aspergillosis
  2. Bronchocentric granulomatosis
III. Eosinophilic lung disease associated with angiitis and/or granulomatosis
 A. Wegener's granulomatosis
 B. Allergic granulomatosis
 C. Polyarteritis nodosa
 D. Necrotizing alveolitis
 E. Necrotizing "sarcoidal" angiitis and granulomatosis

Modified from: Fraser, R.G.; Pare, J.A.: *Diagnosis of Diseases of the Chest*, 2nd ed., Vol. 2, Saunders Co., 1978, p. 901.

VII-12 DIFFERENTIAL DIAGNOSIS OF PULMONARY INTERSTITIAL DISEASE

I. Idiopathic
   A. Idiopathic hemosiderosis
   B. Pulmonary alveolar proteinosis
II. Environmental dusts and chemical fumes
   A. Silica
   B. Asbestos
   C. Sugar cane
   D. Tall
   E. Coal dust
   F. Beryllium
   G. Chemical fumes
      1. Nitrogen dioxine
      2. Chlorine, ammonia, sulfur dioxide
III. Drugs
   A. Sulfonamides
   B. Chlorothiazide
   C. Bleomycin
   D. Busulfan
   E. N-nitroso-N-methylurethane
   F. Nitrofurantoin
   G. Gold salts
IV. Infection
   A. Viruses
      1. Influenza
      2. Cytomegalovirus
      3. Varicella
   B. Bacterial I. tuberculosis
   C. Fungal
      1. Histoplasmosis
      2. Coccidioidomycosis
   D. Parasites
      1. Schistosomiasis
      2. Pneumocystis carinii
V. Physical
   A. X-ray irradiation
   B. Atelectasis
   C. Aspiration of lipid
   D. Chronic pulmonary edema
VI. Immunologic
   A. Hypersensitivity pneumonitis (extrinsic allergic alveolitis)
   B. Sarcoid
   C. Rheumatoid lung
   D. Scleroderma
   E. Sjögren's syndrome
   F. Dermatomyositis
   G. Systemic lupus erythematosus

VII-12 DIFFERENTIAL DIAGNOSIS OF PULMONARY INTERSTITIAL DISEASE (CONTINUED)

VII. Neoplastic
- A. Lymphangitic carcinoma
- B. Histiocytosis-X

VIII. Circulatory
- A. Thromboemboli
  1. Pulmonary emboli
- B. Congestive heart failure

Modified from: Turino, G.M.: in *Pulmonary Diseases and Disorders*, Fishman, A.P. (ed.), Vol. 1, McGraw-Hill Book Company, New York, 1980, p. 726.

VII-13 DIFFERENTIAL DIAGNOSIS OF RESPIRATORY FAILURE

I. Pulmonary origin
- A. Diffuse obstructive airway disease
- B. Central airway obstruction
- C. Restrictive lung disease
- D. Pulmonary vascular disease
  1. Pulmonary embolus
  2. Arteriovenous fistula
- E. Pleural and chest wall disease
  1. Pleural effusions
  2. Pleural fibrosis
  3. Pneumothorax
  4. Flail chest
  5. Fixed chest wall deformities
- F. Diaphragm muscle fatigue

II. Extrapulmonary origin
- A. Neuromuscular disease
- B. Central nervous system disease
- C. Drug suppression of respiratory center
- D. Primary hypoventilation syndromes (sleep apnea syndromes)
  1. Central type
  2. Obstructive
  3. Mixed
- E. Laryngeal obstruction
- F. Congestive heart failure

VII-14 CRITERIA FOR EXTUBATION

I. Vital capacity $> 10\text{-}15$ cc/kg; tidal volume 4-5 cc/kg
II. Peak inspiratory force more negative than -20 cm H_2O
III. P(A-a) O_2 on 100% $IO_2 < 350$ mm Hg
IV. PEEP < 5 cm H_2O
V. $FIOI_2 < 40\%$
VI. Spontaneous ventilation on T-tube > 18 hours with an acceptable arterial pH and paO_2

Modified from: Smith, T.W., et al.: in *Manual of Medical Therapeutics*, Freitag, J.J., Miller, L.W. (eds.), Little, Brown and Company, Boston, 23rd Ed., 1980, p. 157.

VII-15 DIFFERENTIAL DIAGNOSIS OF ALVEOLAR HYPERVENTILATION

I. Increase in stimuli from the periphery
   A. Hypoxia
   B. Diffuse interstitial edema or disease
   C. Pulmonary emboli
   D. Pain
   E. Circulatory collapse
   F. Cooling
   G. Simulated breath sounds
II. Increase in stimuli from central nervous system
   A. Anxiety
   B. Voluntary
   C. Fever
   D. Brainstem lesions
   E. Salicylates
   F. Intracranial hemorrhage
   G. Metabolic acidosis
   H. Descent from altitude
III. Unknown stimuli
   A. Cirrhosis of the liver
   B. Uremia
   C. Pregnancy
IV. Assisted ventilation

Modified from: Fishman, A.P.: in *Pulmonary Diseases and Disorders*, Fishman, A.P. (ed.), Vol. I, McGraw-Hill Book Company, New York, 1980, p. 421.

VII-16 DIFFERENTIAL DIAGNOSIS OF CHRONIC ALVEOLAR HYPOVENTILATION

I. Functional depression of respiratory neurons
  A. Sleep
  B. Hypercapnea
  C. Metabolic alkalosis
  D. Drugs (narcotics, sedatives)
II. Anatomic damage to the central nervous system
  A. Bulbar poliomyelitis
  B. Guillain-Barré syndrome
  C. Encephalitis
  D. Brain stem infarction
  E. Bilateral cervical cordotomy
  F. Pickwickian syndrome
    1. Idiopathic
    2. Central sleep apnea syndromes
III. Neuromuscular disorders affecting chest cage
  A. Poliomyelitis
  B. Myxedema
  C. Myasthenia gravis
  D. Skeletal deformity
  E. Polymyositis
  F. Obesity
IV. Obstruction to upper airways
  A. Peripheral sleep-apnea syndromes
  B. Extrathoracic obstruction
V. Obstructive disease of the airways

Modified from: Fishman, A.P.: in *Pulmonary Diseases and Disorders*, Fishman, A.P. (ed.), Vol. 1, McGraw-Hill Book Company, New York, 1980, p. 422.

VII-17 SYMPTOMS AND SIGNS OBSERVED IN 327 PATIENTS WITH ANGIOGRAPHICALLY DOCUMENTED PULMONARY EMBOLI

Symptoms and signs	(N = 327) %	Massive embolism (N = 197) %	Submassive embolism (N = 130) %
Symptoms			
Chest pain	88	85	89
Pleuritic	74	64	85
Nonpleuritic	14	6	8
Dyspnea	85	85	82
Apprehension	59	65	50
Cough	53	53	52
Hemoptysis	30	23	40
Sweats	27	29	23
Syncope	13	20	6
Signs			
Respirations > 16/min.	92	95	87
Rales	58	57	60
Increased S$_2$P*	53	58	45
Pulse > 100 min.	44	48	38
Temperature > 37.8°C	43	43	42
Diaphoresis	36	42	27
Gallop	34	39	25
Phlebitis	32	36	26
Edema	24	28	25
Murmur	23	27	27
Cyanosis	19	25	9

* Increased S$_2$P = increase in intensity of the pulmonic component of the second heart sound.

Bell, W.R., Simon, T.L., and DeMets, D.L.: The clinical features of submassive and massive pulmonary emboli. Am. J. Med. 62:355, 1977.

VII-18 ECG CHANGES IN PULMONARY EMBOLISM

Normal sinus rhythm or sinus tachycardia	75%-80%
Rhythm changes	20%-25%
Premature atrial contractions	10%
Premature ventricular contractions	10%
Atrial fibrillation	5%
Conduction disturbance	10%
QRS axis changes	
Acute right shift	15%
Right bundle branch block	8%
T changes	40%
Depressed ST segments	25%
Elevated ST segments	16%

* Significantly more common in massive embolism.

Stein, P.D., Dalen, J.E., McIntyre, K.M., Sasahara, A.A., Wenger, N.K., and Willis, P.W.: The electro- cardiogram in acute pulmonary embolism. Progr. Cardiovasc. Dis. 17:247, 1974.

VII-19 COMMON FINDINGS ON CHEST ROENTGENOGRAM IN PULMONARY EMBOLISM

Elevated diaphragm	40% - 60%
Pleural effusion	30%
Infiltrate or consolidation	40%
Atelectasis	20%
Pulmonary vessel changes	40%
Changes in heart size	10%

Moses, D.L., Silver, T.M., and Bookstein, J.T.: The complementary roles of chest radiography, lung scanning, and selective pulmonary angiography in the diagnosis of pulmonary embolism.

VII-20 CAUSES OF NON-CARDIAC PULMONARY EDEMA

    I. High altitude pulmonary edema
    II. Opiate induced
    III. Neurogenic pulmonary edema
    IV. Pneumonia
    V. Drugs/toxins
        A. Ethchlorvynol
        B. Paraquat
        C. Phosgene
        D. Hydrogen chloride
        E. Ammonia
        F. Mercury vapor
        G. Nitrogen oxides
        H. Sulfuroxides
        I. Parathion
    VI. Blood transfusion mismatch
    VII. Shock
    VIII. Trauma

Adapted from: Overland, E.S., and Severinghaus, J.W.: Noncardiac Pulmonary Edema, in *Advances in Internal Medicine*, Vol. 23, 1978, pp. 307-326.

VII-21 PROGNOSTIC INDICATORS IN PNEUMOCOCCAL PNEUMONIA

    I. Multilobe involvement (hypoxia)
    II. Metastatic sites of infection such as bone, pericardium, meningitis (positive blood cultures)
    III. Immunocompromised states (Hodgkin's & non-Hodgkin's lymphoma, leukemia, corticosteroid use)
    IV. Asplenic states (sickle cell anemia, post-splenectomy)
    V. Capsular serotype (types 3)
    VI. WBC < 5000 or > 25,000
    VII. Extremes of age (young & old) < 1 or > 55
    VIII. Complement abnormalities
    IX. Agammaglobulinemia
    X. Pre-existing illnesses (chronic lung disease, diabetes mellitus)
    XI. Ethanolism

VII-22 CAUSES OF LUNG ABSCESS

   I. Necrotizing infections
      A. Pyogenic bacteria (Staph., Klebsiella, Strep., Bacteroides, Fusobacterium, Nocardia, Anaerobic and Microaerophilic Cocci and Streptococci, other anaerobes)
      B. Mycobacterium
      C. Fungi (histoplasmosis, coccidioidomycosis)
      D. Parasitic (ameba, lung flukes)
  II. Cavitary Infarction
      A. Bland embolism
      B. Septic embolism
      C. Vasculitis
 III. Cavitary Malignancy
      A. Primary bronchogenic
      B. Metastatic (uncommon for these to cavitate)
  IV. Miscellaneous
      A. Infected cysts
      B. Necrotic lesions (silicosis, Caplan's, coal miner's pneumoconiosis)

Modified From: Hirschmann, J.V., et al., *Harrison's Principles of Internal Medicine*, McGraw Hill Book Co., New York City, 9th Edition, 1980, pg. 1228.

VII-23 CRITERIA FOR THE DIAGNOSIS OF ALLERGIC BRONCHOPULMONARY ASPERGILLOSIS

   I. Primary
      A. Asthma
      B. Peripheral blood and sputum eosinophilia
      C. Positive immediate skin test
      D. Positive serum precipitins
      E. Elevated IgE levels
      F. Recurrent pulmonary infiltrates
      G. Central bronchiectasis on bronchograms
  II. Secondary
      A. Aspergillus in sputum on repeated culture
      B. Expectoration of "brown plugs"
      C. Positive 6-8 hour delayed skin test

Note: The first six primary signs should be present for the diagnosis to be made.

Corrigan, K., Kory, R.: Diagnosis and Management of Pulmonary Aspergillosis. Ann. Int. Med. 86:405, 1977.

VII-24 PULMONARY COMPLICATIONS OF DIALYSIS

I. Peritoneal dialysis
   A. Elevation of diaphragm with decrease of vital capacity
   B. Basilar atelectasis with or without pneumonitis
   C. Pleural effusion
II. Hemodialysis
   A. Pulmonary embolization (septic and sterile)
   B. Air embolism
   C. Cardiac failure with pulmonary edema
   D. Sequestration of leukocytes in the lung

Modified from: Edelman, N.H.: in *Pulmonary Diseases and Disorders*, Fishman, A.P. (ed.), Vol. 2, McGraw-Hill Book Company, New York, 1980, p. 1353.

VII-25 PARANEOPLASTIC SYNDROMES ASSOCIATED WITH BRONCHOGENIC CARCINOMA

I. Metabolic and endocrine
   A. Gynecomastia
   B. Cushing's syndrome (hypokalemic alkalosis)
   C. SIADH
      1. Hyponatremia
   D. Hypercalcemia
      1. Metabolic
      2. Pseudohyperparathyroidism with increased PTH levels
      3. Elaboration of prostaglandins
      4. Elaboration of vitamin D bile sterols
   E. Carcinoid disorders
II. Neuromuscular disorders
   A. Myasthenic syndrome (Eaton-Lambert)
   B. Peripheral neuropathy—motor/sensory/mixed
   C. Cerebellar degeneration
III. Connective tissue disorders
   A. Clubbing of digits
   B. Pulmonary hypertrophic osteoarthropathy
   C. Dermatomyositis - polymyositis
   D. Acanthosis nigricans
IV. Vascular disorders
   A. Thrombophlebitis
   B. Thromboctopenic purpura
   C. Thrombocythemia
   D. Marantic endocarditis

Carr, David T., Rosenow, Edward C.: Bronchogenic carcinoma. Basics of Respiratory Diseases, vol. 5, no. 5, May, 1977.

VII-26 DIFFERENTIAL DIAGNOSIS OF A SOLITARY PULMONARY NODULE

I. Malignant neoplasm (40%)
   A. Primary lung carcinoma or sarcoma
   B. Metastatic carcinoma or sarcoma
II. Inflammation (40%)
   A. Granulomas
   B. Inflammatory pseudotumor
   C. Localized scar
III. Benign neoplasms (20%)
   A. "Hamartoma"
   B. Other mesenchymal tumors
   C. Clear cell ("sugar") tumor
IV. Malformation
   A. Pulmonary sequestration
   B. Pulmonary arteriovenous fistula

Modified from: Ochs, R.N.: in *Pulmonary Diseases and Disorders*, Fishman, A.P. (ed.), Vol. 2, McGraw-Hill Book Company, New York, 1980, p. 1444.

VII-27 DIFFERENTIAL DIAGNOSIS OF TUMORS METASTATIC TO THE LUNGS

I. Parenchymal nodules
- A. Solitary carcinoma
  1. Large bowel
  2. Breast
  3. Kidney
  4. Female genital tract
  5. Skin
- B. Solitary sarcoma
  1. Osteogenic
- C. Multiple nodules
  1. Any carcinoma
  2. Any sarcoma

II. Endobronchial metastases
- A. Carcinoma
  1. Kidney
  2. Large bowel
- B. Fibrosarcoma
- C. Malignant melanoma

III. Lymphangitic metastases (carcinomas)
- A. Lung
- B. Stomach
- C. Breast
- D. Large bowel
- E. Pancreas

Modified from: Ochs, R.N.: in *Pulmonary Diseases and Disorders*, Fishman, A.P. (ed.), Vol. 2, McGraw-Hill Book Company, New York, 1980, p. 1447.

VII-28 DIFFERENTIAL DIAGNOSIS OF A MEDIASTINAL MASS

I. Situated predominantly in the anterior compartment
  A. Thymoma
  B. Germ cell neoplasm
    1. Teratoma
    2. Seminoma
    3. Primary choriocarcinoma
    4. Endodermal sinus tumor
  C. Thyroid masses
  D. Parathyroid masses
  E. Mesenchymal neoplasms
    1. Lipoma
    2. Fibroma
    3. Hemangioma
    4. Lymphangioma
II. Situated predominantly in the middle compartment
  A. Lymph node enlargement caused by lymphoma or leukemia
  B. Lymph node enlargement caused by metastatic carcinoma
  C. Lymph node enlargement caused by infections
    1. Fungal
    2. Tuberculosis
    3. Mononucleosis
  D. Primary tracheal neoplasms
  E. Brochogenic cyst
  F. Masses situated in the anterior cardiophrenic angle
    1. Pleuropericardial (mesothelial) cysts
    2. Hernia through the foramen of Morgagni
    3. Enlargement of diaphragmatic lymph nodes
    4. Pericardial fat necrosis
  G. Dilatation of the main pulmonary artery
  H. Dilatation of the major mediastinal veins
  I. Dilatation of the aorta or its branches

III. Situated predominantly in the posterior compartment
  A. Neurogenic neoplasms
  B. Meningocele
  C. Neurenteric cysts
  D. Gastroenteric cysts
  E. Thoracic duct cysts
  F. Primary lesions of the esophagus
    1. Neoplasm
    2. Diverticula
    3. Megaesophagus
    4. Hiatal hernia
  G. Hernia through the foramen of Bochdalek
  H. Diseases of the thoracic spine
    1. Neoplasms
    2. Infectious spondylitis
    3. Fracture with hematoma
  I. Extramedullary hematopoiesis

Adapted from: Fraser, R.G.; Pare, J.A.: *Diagnosis of Diseases of the Chest*, second ed., Vol. III, 1979, p. 1793.

VIII—Clinical Immunology & Rheumatology

VIII-1 DIAGNOSTIC CRITERIA FOR SYSTEMIC LUPUS ERYTHEMATOSUS

    I. Malar rash
   II. Discoid lupus
  III. Photosensitivity
  IV. Oral ulcers
   V. Arthritis
  VI. Proteinuria (> 0.5 g/day) or cellular casts
 VII. Seizures or psychosis
VIII. Pleuritis or pericarditis
  IX. One of the following
     A. Hemolytic anemia
     B. Leukopenia
     C. Thrombocytopenia
   X. One of the following
     A. Antibody to DNA
     B. Antibody to SM
     C. LE cells
  XI. Positive fluorescence antinuclear antibody

Four or more are required for the diagnosis of systemic lupus erythematosus.

Eng, M.T., et al. Proposed revised criteria, 1982 Arthritis and Rheumatism 25:4; 2, 1982.

VIII-2 DIFFERENTIAL DIAGNOSIS OF RAYNAUD'S PHENOMENON

I. Primary - Idiopathic
II. Secondary
  A. Collagen vascular disease
    1. Scleroderma (80-90%)
    2. Systemic lupus erythematosus (10-35%)
    3. Rheumatoid arthritis
    4. Systemic vasculitis
    5. Polymyositis (25%)
  B. Traumatic vasospastic disease
  C. Peripheral vascular disease
  D. Nerve compression
    1. Thoracic outlet obstruction
    2. Carpal tunnel syndrome
  E. Drugs and chemicals
    1. Ergot alkaloids
    2. Methysergide
    3. Polyvinyl chloride
    4. Beta blockers
    5. Bleomycin
  F. Hematologic abnormalities
    1. Cryoglobulinemia
    2. Cold agglutinin and disease
    3. Polycythemia
    4. Macroglobulinemia
  G. Miscellaneous
    1. Hepatitis
    2. Malignancy

Adapted from: Crow, M., Manual of Rheumatology and Outpatient Orthopedic Disorders, Little Brown, Boston, 1981, p. 72.

VIII-3 POLYMYALGIA RHEUMATICA

I. Diagnostic Criteria
   A. Musculoskeletal pain in neck, shoulders, and pelvic girdle for at least one month
   B. Patients usually at least 60 years of age
   C. Elevated ESR (usually greater than 50)
   D. Frequently present
      1. Anemia
      2. Headache

II. Differential Diagnosis
   A. Connective tissue disorders
      1. Rheumatoid arthritis
      2. Polymyositis
      3. Vasculitis
      4. Lupus erythematosus
   B. Neoplastic disorders
      1. Multiple myeloma
      2. Occult tumors
   C. Infections
      1. Post viral syndromes (esp. influenza)
      2. Occult infection
   D. Miscellaneous
      1. Degenerative joint disease
      2. Fibromyalgia

VIII-4 CRITERIA FOR DIAGNOSIS

Stevens-Johnson Syndrome

I. Major Criteria
  A. Skin lesions
  B. Erythema multiforme exudativum
  C. Stomatitis (ulcerative)
  D. Genital or anal ulcers
II. Minor Criteria
  A. Pneumonitis - preceding or coexistent
  B. History of upper respiratory or genitourinary infection treated with sulfonamides or antibiotics
  C. Arthralgias
  D. Conjunctivitis
  E. History of ingestion of wide variety of drugs, both prescription and nonprescription

Adapted from: Ehrlich, G.: in *Arthritis and Allied Conditions*, J.L. Hollander and D.J. McCarty (Eds.), Philadelphia, Lea & Febiger, 1979, p. 677.

VIII-5 DIAGNOSIS OF BEHÇET'S SYNDROME

  I. Major criteria:
    A. Mouth (aphthous) ulcers
    B. Iritis (with hypopyon)
    C. Genital ulcers
    D. Skin lesions
      1. Pyoderma
      2. Nodose lesions
 II. Minor criteria:
    A. Arthritis
      1. Of major joints
      2. Arthralgias
    B. Vascular disease
      1. Migratory superficial phlebitis
      2. Major vessel thrombosis
      3. Aneurysms
      4. Peripheral gangrene
      5. Retinal and vitreous hemorrhage, papilledema
    C. Central nervous system disease
      1. Brain stem syndrome
      2. Meningomyelitis
      3. Confusional states
    D. Gastrointestinal disease
      1. Malabsorption
      2. Colonic ulcers
      3. Dilated intestinal loops
    E. Epididymitis

Adapted from: Ehrlich, G.: in *Arthritis and Allied Conditions*, J.L. Hollander and D.J. McCarty (Eds.), Philadelphia, Lea & Febiger, 1979, p. 676.

VIII-6 CRITERIA FOR THE DIAGNOSIS OF SCLERODERMA

(Progressive Systemic Sclerosis)

    I. Single major criterion - proximal scleroderma*
   II. Minor criteria
      A. Sclerodactyly
      B. Digital pitting of finger tips
      C. Bibasilar pulmonary fibrosis

* A term indicating bilateral and symmetric sclerodermatous changes in any area proximal to the metacarpal or metatarsal phalangeal joints.

The diagnosis of definite scleroderma can be made with 1 major or 2 or more minor criteria.

Source: Bull. Rheum. Dis. 31:1-6, 1981.

VIII-7 DIAGNOSTIC CRITERIA FOR POLYMYOSITIS/DERMATOMYOSITIS

    I. Symmetric proximal muscle weakness
   II. Characteristic EMG abnormalities
  III. Characteristic abnormalities upon histologic examination of muscle biopsy specimens
  IV. Elevation of serum enzymes (CPK, SGOT, LDH, Aldolase)
   V. Characteristic skin rash
      A. Polymyositis -
         1. Definite - 4 criteria present
         2. Probable - 3 criteria present
         3. Possible - 2 criteria present
      B. Dermatomyositis - must have characteristic rash
         1. Definite - 3 or 4 criteria present
         2. Probable - 2 criteria present
         3. Possible - I criteria present

Modified from: Polk, R.: Manual of Rheumatology and Outpatient Orthopedic Disorders, Little, Brown and Co., Boston, 1981, pp. 221-222.

VIII-8 RHEUMATOID ARTHRITIS DIAGNOSTIC CRITERIA

    I. Morning stiffness>45 minutes.

    II. Pain on motion or tenderness in at least one joint.*

    III. Swelling (soft tissue thickening or fluid, not bony overgrowth alone) in at least one joint.*

    IV. Swelling of at least one other joint.*†

    V. Symmetrical joint swelling with simultaneous involvement of the same joint on both sides of the body.*† Terminal phalangeal joint involvement will not satisfy the criterion.

    VI. Subcutaneous nodules over bony prominences, on extensor surfaces, or in juxta-articular regions.*

    VII. Roentgenographic changes typical of rheumatoid arthritis (which must include at least bony decalcification localized to or greatest around the involved joints and not just degenerative changes).†

    VIII. Positive agglutination (anti-gammaglobulin) test.†

    IX. Poor mucin precipitate from synovial fluid (with shreds and cloudy solution).

    X. Characteristic histologic changes in synovial membrane.†

    XI. Characteristic histologic changes in nodules.†

* Observed by a physician.

Categories	Number of Criteria required	Minimum Duration of Continuous Symptoms
Classic	7 of 11	Six weeks (Nos 1-5)
Definite	5 of 11	Six weeks (Nos 1-5)
Probable	3 of 11	Six weeks (one of Nos 1-5)

Exclusions†

   I. The typical rash of disseminated lupus erythematosus.
  II. High concentration of lupus erythematosus cells.
 III. Histologic evidence of periarteritis nodosa.
 IV. Weakness of neck, trunk, and pharyngeal muscles or persistent muscle swelling or dermatomyositis.
  V. Definite scleroderma.
 VI. Clinical picture characteristic of rheumatic fever.
VII. Clinical picture characteristic of gouty arthritis.
VIII. Tophi.
 IX. Clinical picture characteristic of acute infectious arthritis.
  X. Tubercle bacilli in the joints or histologic evidence of joint tuberculosis.
 XI. Clinical picture characteristic of Reiter's syndrome.
XII. Clinical picture characteristic of the shoulder-hand syndrome.
XIII. Clinical picture characteristic of hypertrophic pulmonary osteoarthropathy.
XIV. Clinical picture characteristic of neuroarthropathy.
 XV. Homogentisic acid in the urine detectable grossly with alkalinization.
XVI. Histologic evidence of sarcoid or positive Kveim test.
XVII. Multiple myeloma.
XVIII. Characteristic skin lesions of erythema nodosum.
XIX. Leukemia or lymphoma.
 XX. Agammaglobulinemia.

Ropes, M.W. et al.: Bull. Rheum. Dis. 9:175-197, 1958.

VIII-9 DIAGNOSTIC CRITERIA FOR JUVENILE RHEUMATOID ARTHRITIS

Due to diagnostic difficulty the Arthritis Foundation adopted the following criteria expanding Ansell and Bywaters criteria in 1972.

I. Classification for Juvenile rheumatoid arthritis (JRA).*
   A. Polyarthritis (2 or more joints) or monoarticular arthritis of more than 3 months duration. Any diagnosis listed under exclusions eliminates JRA from consideration. Swelling of a joint must be present to fulfill criteria or 2 of 3 features (a. heat, b. pain and tenderness, c. limitation of motion) must be present.
   B. Polyarthritis present for more than 6 weeks but less than 3 months should require one of the following manifestations for diagnosis.
      1. Rash of rheumatoid arthritis.
      2. Positive rheumatoid factor.
      3. Iridocyclitis.
      4. Cervical vertebral involvement.
      5. Pericarditis.
      6. Tenosynovitis.
      7. Intermittent fever.
      8. Morning stiffness.
II. Exclusions
   A. Rheumatic fever.
   B. Connective tissue diseases i.e. SLE, PSS, dermatomyositis.
   C. Infectious disease i.e. pyogenic arthritis, sepsis, viral diseases, tuberculosis, syphilis, fungal diseases.
   D. Allergic reactions.
   E. Anaphylactoid purpura.
   F. Ulcerative colitis and regional enteritis.
   G. Neoplastic disease i.e. lymphoma, leukemia.
   H. Hematologic disorders i.e. sickle cell anemia, hemophilia, thalassemia.
   I. Trauma.
   J. Miscellaneous diseases i.e. Reiter's syndrome, sarcoidosis gammaglobulinemia, hypertrophic osteoarthropathy, ankylosing spondylitis, villonodular synovitis, Gaucher's disease, mucopolysaccharidases, and bone dysplasia.

*Source: The Arthritis Foundation.

VIII-10   DIAGNOSTIC CRITERIA OF ANKYLOSING SPONDYLITIS

    I. Low back pain of over three months' duration, unrelieved by rest.
    II. Pain and stiffness in the thoracic cage.
    III. Limited chest expansion.
    IV. Limited motion in the lumbar spine.
    V. Past or present evidence of iritis.
    VI. Bilateral radiographic sacroiliitis.
    VII. Radiographic syndesmophytosis.

Diagnosis requires four of the five clinical criteria or No. 6 and one other criterion.

Adapted from: Ehrlich, G.: in *Arthritis and Allied Conditions*, J.L. Hollander and D.J. McCarty (Eds.), Philadelphia, Lea & Febiger, 1979, p. 621.

VIII-11   CRITERIA FOR DIAGNOSIS OF GOUTY ARTHRITIS

A patient with six or more variable positive would be classified as having gout.

    I. Monoarticulr arthritis
    II. Occurrence of more than one attack
    III. Maximal inflammation developing within one day
    IV. Redness over joints
    V. Pain or swelling in the first metatarsophalangeal joint
    VI. Unilateral involvement of (5)
    VII. Unilateral involvement of a tarsal joint
    VIII. Tophus--either proved or suspected to contain MSU crystals
    IX. Serum uric acid>normal for that particular lab
    X. X-ray demonstrated asymmetric joint swelling
    XI. Subcortical cysts without erosions on x-ray
    XII. Monosodium urate crystals in joint fluid
    XIII. Joint fluid negative for organisms

Synovial fluid MSU crystals or proved tophus are universally accepted as the ultimate diagnosis for gout.

American Rheumatism Association, July 1975.

VIII-12 PROVISIONAL CRITERIA FOR DIAGNOSIS OF PSORIATIC ARTHRITIS*

I. Mandatory

Clinically apparent psoriasis (skin or nails) in association with pain and soft tissue swelling and/or limitation of motion in at least one joint, observed by a physician for six weeks or longer.

II. Supportive

A. Pain and soft tissue swelling and/or limitation of motion in one or more other joints, observed by a physician.

B. Presence of an inflammatory arthritis in distal interphalangeal joint.

C. Specific exclusions--Heberden's or Bouchard's nodes.

D. Presence of "sausage" fingers or toes.

E. An asymmetric distribution of the arthritis in the hands and feet.

F. Absence of subcutaneous nodules.

G. A negative test for rheumatoid factor in the serum.

H. An inflammatory synovial fluid with a normal or increased C3 or C4 level, and an absence of: (a) infection, including AFB, (b) crystals of monosodium urate or calcium pyrophosphate.

I. A synovial biopsy showing synovial lining hypertrophy with a predominantly mononuclear cell infiltration, and an absence of: (a) granuloma formation, (b) tumor.

J. Peripheral radiographs showing an erosive arthritis of small joints with a relative lack of osteoporosis. Specific exclusion--erosive osteoarthritis.

K. Axial radiographs showing one or more of the following: (a) sacroiliitis, (b) syndesmophytes (sometimes atypical), and (c) paravertebral ossification.

* Definite psoriatic arthritis--mandatory plus six supportive criteria. Probable psoriatic arthritis--mandatory plus four supportive criteria. Possible psoriatic arthritis--mandatory plus two supportive criteria.

Adapted from: Bennett, R.: in *Arthritis and Allied Conditions*, Hollander, J.C., Mc Carty, D.E. (Eds.), Lea & Febiger, Philadelphia, 1979, p. 645.

VIII-13 DIFFERENTIAL DIAGNOSIS OF INFLAMMATORY MONOARTHRITIS

   I. Crystal induced
      A. Gout
      B. Pseudogout
      C. Calcific tendinitis
  II. Palindromic rheumatism
 III. Infectious arthritis
      A. Septic
      B. Tubercular
      C. Fungal
      D. Viral
 IV. Other
      A. Tendinitis
      B. Bursitis
      C. Juvenile rheumatoid arthritis

Modified from: McCarty, D.: in *Arthritis and Allied Conditions*, J.L. Hollander and D.J. McCarty (Eds.), Philadelphia, Lea & Febiger, 1979, p. 47.

VIII-14 DIAGNOSTIC FEATURES OF SARCOIDOSIS

I. Sarcoidosis
   A. Noncaseating granulomas on biopsy. Must exclude other causes of granulomas.
   B. Hilar and right paratracheal adenopathy in 90%.
   C. Skin lesions, uveitis, or involvement of almost any tissue.
   D. Onset most often in third and fourth decades, but cases reported at all ages.
   E. Impaired delayed hypersensitivity in 85%.
   F. Frequent hyperglobulinemia.

II. Sarcoid arthropathy
   Acute Sarcoidosis (Lofgren's Syndrome)
   A. Often periarticular and very tender, warm swelling.
   B. Ankles and knees almost invariably involved.
   C. May be initial manifestation.
   D. Joint motion may be normal.
   E. Synovial effusions infrequent and usually mildly inflammatory when present.
   F. Usually nonspecific mild synovitis on synovial biopsy.
   G. Self-limited in weeks to 4 months.

III. Chronic Sarcoidosis
   A. May be acute and evanescent, recurrent or chronic.
   B. Noncaseating granulomas more commonly demonstrable in synovium.
   C. Usually nondestructive despite chronic or recurrent disease.

Adapted from: Schumacher, H.: in *Arthritis and Allied Conditions*, J.L. Hollander and D.J. McCarty (Eds.), Philadelphia, Lea & Febiger, 1979, p. 923.

VIII-15 DIFFERENTIAL DIAGNOSIS OF POSITIVE BLOOD TEST FOR RHEUMATOID FACTOR

I. Rheumatologic disease
   A. Rheumatoid arthritis
   B. Juvenile rheumatoid arthritis
   C. Systemic lupus erythematosus
   D. Mixed connective tissue disease
   E. Behçet's syndrome
   F. Sjögren's syndrome
II. Infectious disease
   A. Bacterial (especially endocarditis)
   B. Syphilis
   C. Viral hepatitis
   D. Parasitic infections
   E. Granulomatous disease
   F. Mononucleosis
III. Pulmonary disease
   A. Bronchitis or asthma
   B. Coal miner's disease
   C. Asbestosis
   D. Idiopathic pulmonary fibrosis
   E. Sarcoidosis
IV. Other diseases
   A. Cirrhosis
   B. Myocardial infarction
   C. Neoplasms
V. Healthy Persons - Increases with age

Modified from: Coffey, R., et al., Postgraduate Medicine 70:164, 1981.

VIII-16 CRYOGLOBULINEMIA

I. Essential or idiopathic
II. Secondary to or associated with
   A. Hemopoietic disorders
      1. Multiple myeloma
      2. Waldenström's macroglobulinemia
      3. Lymphatic leukemia, lymphosarcoma
      4. Polycythemia vera
      5. Sickle cell anemia
   B. Connective tissue disorders
      1. Systemic lupus erythematosus
      2. Syndrome of arthralgia, purpura, nephritis, and weakness
      3. Rheumatoid arthritis
      4. Ankylosing spondylitis
      5. Polyarteritis nodosa
      6. Sjögren's syndrome
      7. Thyroiditis
      8. Lymphoepithelial tumors of parotid gland
      9. Acute poststreptococcal glomerulonephritis
   C. Chronic infections
      1. Subacute bacterial endocarditis
      2. Visceral leishmaniasis (kala-azar)
      3. Syphilis
      4. Toxoplasmosis
      5. Leprosy
   D. Others
      1. Chronic liver disease (cirrhosis, cholecystitis, chronic hepatitis, gallbladder neoplasm)
      2. Skin disorders (porphyria cutanea tarda, pemphigus, erythrodermia)
      3. Acute myocardial infarction
      4. Infectious mononucleosis
      5. Ulcerative colitis
      6. Sarcoidosis
      7. Cytomegalovirus infection

VIII-17 CLASSIFICATION OF IMMUNE DEFICIENCY STATES

I. Immunoglobulin deficiency
  A. Transient hypogammaglobulinemia of infancy
  B. Infantile X-linked agammaglobulinemia
  C. Common variable hypogammaglobulinemia
  D. Dysgammaglobulinemia (selective IgA deficiency)
  E. Acquired hypogammaglobulinemia
    1. Decreased synthesis - lymphoreticular disease
    2. Increased catabolism - nephrotic syndrome
    3. Increased loss - exudative enteropathy, burns, nephrosis
    4. Increased synthesis of abnormal Ig - multiple myeloma
II. Cell-mediated immunity deficiency
  A. Congenital thymic aplasia (DiGeorge syndrome)
  B. Small lymphocyte depletion
    1. Thoracic duct drainage
    2. Intestinal lymphangiectasia
  C. Functional lymphocyte deficiency
    1. Viral infection
    2. Granulomatous disease
  D. Mediator deficiency (e.g. mucocutaneous candidiasis)
III. Combined immunoglobulin and cell-mediated deficiency
   (Severe combined deficiency)

Source: Abdou, Nabih - personal communication.

VIII-18 CLASSIFICATION OF VASCULITIDES

I. Polyarteritis nodosa group of systemic necrotizing vasculitis
   A. Classic polyarteritis nodosa
   B. Allergic granulomatosis
   C. Systemic necrotizing vasculitis--"overlap syndrome"
II. Hypersensitivity vasculitis
III. Subgroups of hypersensitivity vasculitis
   A. Serum sickness and serum sickness-like reactions
   B. Henoch-Schönlein purpura
   C. Essential mixed cryoglobulinemia with vasculitis
   D. Vasculitis associated with malignancies
   E. Vasculitis associated with other primary disorders
IV. Wegener's granulomatosis
V. Lymphomatoid granulomatosis
VI. Giant-cell arteritides
   A. Temporal arteritis
   B. Takayasu's arteritis
VII. Thromboangiitis obliterans (Buerger's disease)
VIII. Mucocutaneous lymph node syndrome
IX. Miscellaneous vasculitides

Reference: Fauci, A.S., Ann. Int. Med. 89:662, 1978.

VIII-19 AUTOANTIBODIES IN SLE

I. To nuclear antigens
   A. Deoxyribonucleic acid
   B. Histones
   C. Nucleoprotein
   D. Nonhistone (acidic) proteins
II. To cytoplasmic antigens
   A. RNA
   B. Ribosomes and other RNA-protein complexes
   C. Cytoplasmic protein and lipid antigens
III. To cell surface antigens
   A. Red cell surface antigens
   B. Granulocyte cell surface antigens
   C. Lymphocyte cell surface antigens
   D. Platelet antigens
IV. To miscellaneous antigens
   A. Clotting factors (lupus anticoagulants)
   B. Synthetic RNA
   C. Tissue-specific (thyroid, liver, muscle, stomach, adrenal)

From: Advances in Internal Medicine, Vol. 26, p. 468, 1980.

VIII-20 PUTATIVE ASSOCIATIONS OF CPPD CRYSTAL DEPOSITION

  I. Group A (true association - high probability)
- A. Hyperparathyroidism
- B. Hemochromatosis
- C. Hemosiderosis
- D. Hypophosphatasia
- E. Hypomagnesemia
- F. Hypothyroidism
- G. Gout
- H. Neuropathic joints
- I. Aging

  II. Group B (true association - modest probability)
- A. Hyperthyroidism
- B. Renal stone
- C. Ankylosing hyperostosis
- D. Ochronosis
- E. Wilson's disease
- F. Hemophilia arthritis

  III. Group C (true association - unlikely)
- A. Diabetes mellitus
- B. Hypertension
- C. Mild azotemia
- D. Hyperuricemia
- E. Gynecomastia
- F. Inflammatory bowel disease
- G. Rheumatoid arthritis
- H. Paget's disease of bone
- I. Acromegaly

(CPPD = calcium pyrophosphate dihydrate.)

IX—Neurology

IX-1 DIFFERENTIAL DIAGNOSIS OF COMA

I. Diseases causing no focal or lateralizing neurologic signs or alterations in cellular content cerebrospinal fluid
   A. Intoxications
      Opiates, barbiturates, tricyclic antidepressants, ethanol
   B. Metabolic disturbances
      Diabetic acidosis, hyperosmolar non-ketotic coma, alcoholic ketoacidosis, uremia, hepatic encephalopathy, hypoxic-hypotensive encephalopathy, hypercapnia, hypoglycemia, hyponatremia, hypernatremic dehydration, hypokalemia, myxedema coma.
   C. Severe systemic infections
   D. Cardiovascular
      Shock, congestive heart failure, hypertensive encephalopathy
   E. Epilepsy
      Post ictal states
II. Diseases causing focal or lateralizing neurologic signs with or without changes in cerebrospinal fluid
   A. Cerebrovascular accidents
      Hemorrhage, thrombosis, embolism
   B. Mass lesions
      Brain tumor, brain abscess
III. Diseases causing meningeal irritation with either blood or pleocytosis in the cerebrospinal fluid, usually without focal or lateralizing signs.
   A. Subarachnoid hemorrhage
      Ruptured aneurysm, A-V malformation, trauma
   B. Meningitis
      Bacterial, fungal
   C. Encephalitis

Modified from: Adams, R.D.: Coma and Related Disturbances of Consciousness in *Harrison's Principles of Internal Medicine*, Isselbacher, K.J., Adams, R.D., Braunwald, E., Petersdorf, R.G., and Wilson, J.D. (eds.), 9th Edition, McGraw-Hill Book Company, New York City, 1980, p. 120.

IX-2 DIFFERENTIAL DIAGNOSIS OF MENINGITIS

I. Bacterial Meningitis
   A. Neisseria meningitidis
   B. Hemophilus influenzae
   C. Streptococcus pneumoniae
   D. Staphylococcus aureus and epidermidis
   E. Gram negatives
      1. Escherichia coli
      2. Klebsiella, proteus, pseudomonas
   F. Mycobacteria
   G. Leptospirosis
   H. Rare
      1. Listeria monocytogenes
      2. Mima-Herellea
II. Viral (Aseptic) Meningitis
   A. Enteroviruses
      1. Coxsackie viruses
      2. Echo viruses
   B. Herpes simplex
      1. Meningitis or meningoencephalitis
   C. Cytomegalovirus
   D. Epstein Barr-virus
   E. Measles
   F. Mumps
   G. Influenza
   H. Varicella zoster
   I. Rubella
   J. Adenovirus
III. Non-viral Agents which may cause encephalitis-aseptic meningitis syndromes
   A. Rickettsial
      1. Rocky Mountain Spotted Fever
      2. Q fever
   B. Chlamydia and mycoplasma
      1. Mycoplasma pneumoniae
      2. Psittacosis

INDEX

Kidney (cont.)